Christ Walk
Crushed

Christ Walk Crushed

A
40-Day
Pilgrimage
toward
Reconciliation

**ANNA FITCH COURIE
and DAVID W. PETERS**

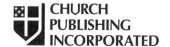

CHURCH
PUBLISHING
INCORPORATED

Unless otherwise noted, the Scripture quotations contained herein are from the New Revised Standard Version Bible, copyright © 1989 by the Division of Christian Education of the National Council of Churches of Christ in the U.S.A. Used by permission. All rights reserved.

Scriptures taken from the Holy Bible, New International Version®, NIV®. Copyright © 1973, 1978, 1984, 2011 by Biblica, Inc.™ Used by permission of Zondervan. All rights reserved worldwide. www.zondervan.com The "NIV" and "New International Version" are trademarks registered in the United States Patent and Trademark Office by Biblica, Inc.™

Scripture quotations marked MSG are taken from *THE MESSAGE*, copyright © 1993, 1994, 1995, 1996, 2000, 2001, 2002 by Eugene H. Peterson. Used by permission of NavPress. All rights reserved. Represented by Tyndale House Publishers, Inc.

Christ Walk™ is a registered trademark of Anna Fitch Courie.

Church Publishing
19 East 34th Street
New York, NY 10016
www.churchpublishing.org

Cover design by Jennifer Kopec, 2Pug Design
Typesetting and page design by Beth Oberholter

Library of Congress Cataloging-in-Publication Data

Names: Fitch Courie, Anna, author. | Peters, David W., author.
Title: Christ walk crushed : a 40-day pilgrimage toward reconciliation / Anna
    Fitch Courie and David W. Peters.
Description: New York, NY : Church Publishing, [2019].
Identifiers: LCCN 2018053221 (print) | LCCN 2019000198 (ebook) | ISBN
    9781640651166 (ebook) | ISBN 9781640651159 (pbk.)
Subjects: LCSH: Reconciliation--Religious aspects--Christianity. | Walking--
    Religious aspects--Christianity. | Health--Religious aspects--Christianity. |
    Spiritual life--Christianity.
Classification: LCC BT738.27 (ebook) | LCC BT738.27 .F58 2019 (print) |
    DDC 248.4/6--dc23
LC record available at https://lccn.loc.gov/2018053221

This book is dedicated to those who suffer in mind, body, or spirit—especially our brothers and sisters in the military and those struggling with disease.

Contents

Appendices

Preface

While I kept silence, my body wasted away
  through my groaning all day long.
For day and night your hand was heavy upon me;
  my strength was dried up as by the heat of summer.
Then I acknowledged my sin to you,
  and I did not hide my iniquity;
I said, "I will confess my transgressions to the LORD,"
  and you forgave the guilt of my sin. —Psalm 32:3–5

Me: Hey God?
God: Yes?
Me: What's the worst thing I could do?
God: Technically, its already been done, and I'm not sure
  it was all that bad.

Grief and suffering are a part of the human condition. I don't think people get through life without experiencing something that makes them pause, wonder, and question their beliefs. These events in life can pull us farther from God as well as bring us closer to understanding God's divine plan in our lives. Whether we are far from God, or God feels close to us, God is always there. However, when people experience suffering, God can feel very far away. Often, we are very angry with God. Sometimes we believe God does not exist. Trauma has a way of doing all of this to us because it feels like the rug has been pulled from under us. It stops us in our tracks. It paralyzes us. It shocks us. Shock has a way of thrusting us into situations that feel so far outside our locus of control we have no idea how to cope. Suffering, pain, distress, damage to our bodies and psyches all have ways of uncovering questions about the Divine that we typically don't address in everyday life.

That's why we've created *Christ Walk Crushed*. There isn't a roadmap on finding your way back to God after events rock your world. When we sat down to write *Christ Walk Crushed,* we wanted to go on a journey with people who, like us, experienced deep loss and needed to find a way back to who they truly were as beloved children of God. We found our way through reconciliation—with ourselves and with God.

We have experienced events in life that caused us to curse God, turn away from and question our faith, and dabble in practices that weren't good for our health or well-being. We discovered that part of our process of becoming reconciled occurred through physical activity. For Anna, the image of the steps we take on a journey was a powerful one that she held in her mind while she was lost and looking for God again. As a nurse she knew that physical exercise in of itself is a powerful way to deal with the stress, anxiety, fear, and frustration that grief and suffering give us. For David, it is a daily journey looking back when he felt truly crushed. We may not understand the events of our lives in the here and the now, but the road stretches ahead where we can continue to take steps towards deeper understanding. The journey gives *purpose* to events outside of our control.

With *Christ Walk Crushed,* we want you to go on that journey with us. Over the next forty days, we'll ask you to pick a route from the Bible that speaks to you (see Appendix A on page 164) and commit to running, walking, biking, or swimming (essentially whatever exercise you want to choose) the miles to complete that biblical route. We want you to come with us and digest each day as a step towards finding your way back to God.

You aren't alone on this journey; here with you each day, David and Anna take turns talking to you and walking with you on the steps towards reconciliation with God. Perhaps you will also find your way back to a local church or minister who may help you find yourself closer to God than when you started out. It may take you several times to start, stop, backtrack, and then move forward on this journey, but most of all we hope that you never stop moving. We want you to know that no matter what, God does love you, there is purpose to this life even in the middle of what has impacted you, and that what you are experiencing now is not the end of the story.

Come. . . take a walk with us.

Anna and David

Acknowledgments

This is my third Christ Walk ™ book, and my sixth title overall. I have learned so much along the way about God, myself, and writing. I've learned that while I am the author, a book is the product of love from a community of believers. These believers make a book happen. I want to thank so many people. For my family and friends who keep telling me to write. For my editor, Sharon, who has worked with me through four books now and knows my horrible writing habits. I am hopeful she is up for number five. For Ryan, who brings each of my books through production; I always seem to forget to say thank you—really, you've taken each of my books to the next level. For Patton and Merryn, who think it's really cool to have a mom that's a writer and are very forgiving for those times I'm off in another world of words. For Treb, who had no idea he married a crazy author twenty years ago and sticks with me anyway. For each and every person who has shared their journey of heartbreak, who has yearned for closeness with God and wasn't sure where to find God, this book is an acknowledgement of that pain, loss, and suffering. There is hope. Finally, I must always acknowledge God, who prods me to write and reminds me daily that if my words touch one person, then the time was well spent. These words might not be the story I intended when once upon a time I dreamed of being a writer, but they were the words God blessed me with. Thanks be to God.

—Anna

I never thought I would write more than one book, mainly because I couldn't imagine a future where I was alive. So much of this book is written with those days in mind—days where it was hard to see a good future—days where I felt crushed. During those difficult days I was helped by both people and books, one of which was a book of daily readings, much like this one, called *Moving Forward: A Devotional Guide for Finding Hope and Peace in the Midst of Divorce* (Hendrickson, 2000) by Jim Smoke. Up until then, I liked to fancy myself as a literary man, a lover of fine books. I was vain about books, always making certain I was seen with the right book. "Daily guide" books are rarely classics, so it was with some reluctance I picked it up, proud man that I was. But then, after a couple of days of reading, I realized it was saving my life. I hope *Christ Walk Crushed* can do this for you. I think it can if you let it. But first, a word of thanks for all those who made my part in this book possible. Thank you to Anna Courie for including me in her brilliant and inspiring series of Christ Walk™ books. I enjoyed her first *Christ Walk* so much and am honored to be part of this family. Many thanks to Sharon Pearson, who could always see the big picture so this book could arrive in your hands. Since this is my first book written after receiving canonical residency in the Diocese of Texas, I want to thank my bishop, The Rt. Rev. C. Andrew Doyle, for equipping me for veterans' ministry and for writing books about the church that have shaped my thinking about how to follow Jesus into the world. Since I first met Anna on an Episcopal Church Foundation-funded trip to Virginia Theological Seminary, I am grateful for ECF and all they do to bring renewal to our church. I wrote most of these words while I wrapped up a twenty-year military career in the U.S. Marine Corps, the Army, and the Army Reserve. Looking back, I cannot enough admire the women and men I served with, especially Kurt Stein, PhD, and those who deployed with me to Baghdad, Iraq, in the 62nd Engineer Battalion from Fort Hood, Texas. A part of me will always be there with them in that place. Lastly I thank God for my wife Sarah Bancroft, a rock star art historian in the art world, the mother of our son, the author of numerous books, and a fictional character in several Daniel Silva novels. Her words of encouragement mean the world to me.

—David

Introduction

What is *Christ Walk Crushed*? It is a spiritual fitness program designed to improve your mind, body, and spiritual health while taking you through a process of reconciliation. By pairing daily meditations with the miles of biblical routes, you will set a physical goal for yourself paired with mental and spiritual exercises. There is a chapter a day (Day 1, Day 2, etc.) to help lift you up spiritually as you make your journey. *Christ Walk Crushed* uses the Christ Walk™ method to engage in a physical mileage goal while meditating on the process of sin, forgiveness, injury, and reconciliation. In many ways, the *Christ Walk Crushed* program seeks to encourage physical action while you process the grief associated with being out of balance in mind, body, and spirit.

In writing this book, we do not claim to be experts on what is the best thing for *you* to do to have a spiritually and physically healthy life. We do not claim to have all the answers. Much like any Christian, we have many questions that we constantly seek answers for, which is an act of faith for each of us individually. We do not claim that this book is the answer to all of the questions that you may have; it is not a diet, nor a guidebook, nor even a recommendation on how you should live. It's a walk to explore those things in your life that you want to work on and process.

After more than ten years of running Christ Walk™ programs at multiple churches, Anna has found that people enjoy having a book as a companion to whatever journey they are on. The book in your hands is that manual/journal for you to have on this interactive experience of the *Christ Walk Crushed* journey. At the end of the forty days, this book should be as much your book as it is ours.

Individuals as well as groups can walk (or run, bike, swim) this journey. The appendices include options for group leaders and options for individuals to transform their *Christ Walk Crushed* experience from journey to journey. There is always another journey, so *Christ Walk Crushed* should not end after one 40-day period. These forty days should transform you to pursue new journeys and new goals.

After completing *Christ Walk Crushed*, you may want to try another of the Christ Walk™ series. It's your choice, just don't stop moving. Our feet are to be used to care for the temple God created within each of us. Keep working on your relationship with God and your relationship with your body, mind, and soul.

If you are physically unable to walk or perform physical exercise, we ask that you look at your life in ways that you can change it and improve it. Everyone has things that they can do to make their life healthier. Perhaps your goal will be to study something new on your journey, pray with more discipline, focus on changing your nutritional habits, or letting go of destructive habits. If you cannot physically exercise, discuss with your health care provider some options that you are willing to do to change. There is a place in this journey for everyone. We may need to be creative on the method that the journey is completed. Pray through those chapters that may not be applicable to you and really focus on the ones that speak to your personal experience. Offering different perspectives and needs, this book may not work for everyone; if you cannot make the journey on your own, consider how you can help others on their journey. At a minimum, keep an open mind and always consider: "What can I do to change?"

How Does This Work?

Through *Christ Walk Crushed*, we have taken our daily journey as members of the Body of Christ and translated that to actual mileage goals that are pulled from routes that Jesus and the disciples took during varying missions. You will find a list of biblical routes (Appendix A) for you to choose a journey to walk, run, bike, pray, volunteer, or whatever activity you choose (the distance of) during the next forty days. Some of these distances are estimates as they are representative of the journeys many in the Bible took as they followed God's call.

We believe God walks with us in every step that we take and the Bible is filled with inspirational guidelines on how to walk with God: mind, body, and spirit. Each day there will be a Bible verse related to a step in the process of reconciliation. It will be paired with a reflection from either David or Anna on that step in the process. We'll close with some questions that we want you to think about or respond to in order to make the journey yours. There will also be a place for you to fill in your steps/distance, activity, feelings for the day, and spiritual thoughts for the day.

Do not rush; this book is designed to be read one chapter a day, with the book as a journal to help you on your way and improve your *Christ Walk Crushed* experience. If at any time you need to change your goals, feel free to do so. Life is a journey with many bumps happening along the way! The challenge is that you continue to have faith on that journey, even if it is in a different way than the one in which you started. If you are doing this as a group, these journal entries may help in everyone sharing their *Christ Walk Crushed* experiences and deepen your understanding of a life of walking with Christ in community. You can use the daily questions to facilitate discussions as a group or use one of the outlines found in the appendices. See Appendix D on page 176 for Recommendations for Groups.

So, how do we measure the steps we took, the distance we travelled? We recommend the purchase of a fitness tracker (Fitbit, Garmin, Apple Watch, Omron, etc.), which can be worn on your wrist or clothing and will track the number of steps/miles travelled each day. Recommendations from the experts encourage every individual to take 10,000 steps a day for heart health. For some, this will be an easy goal and you may want to challenge yourself to more steps. For others, this may be challenging, and you may need to work up to this level of activity. Perhaps this will be one of your goals for the 40-day program. Roughly 2,000–2,500 steps equal a mile. You will track your steps, miles, or time in specific activities towards your overall biblical route. For the purpose of *Christ Walk Crushed*, we generally give one mile for every 2,000 steps. There is a brief description on using a fitness tracker in Appendix B on page 171.

If you want to use another form of exercise other than walking (biking, swimming, aerobics, dance, etc.) you may do that. It takes about fifteen minutes to walk a mile, so every 15-minute block of exercise can be calculated as a mile. It's important to choose an activity that you enjoy and do it; get out there and move, think about every step you take as walking with God. The process of physically moving will help us physically move through the process of reconciliation. It is your walk with Christ, so make it yours. Your job is to give it your best shot with all your heart.

Mileage Calculation Chart

Activity	Time	Steps	Record Miles As:
Walking	15–20 minutes	2,000–2,500	1 or distance on route
Running	Varies	2,000–2,500	Check route distance
Biking	Varies	N/A	Check odometer distance
Aerobics	15 minutes	Varies	1
Dancing	15 minutes	Varies	1
Yoga	15 minutes	Varies	1
Prayer/Meditation	15 minutes	Varies	1
Volunteerism	15 minutes	Varies	1

With *Christ Walk Crushed*, our goal for you is to set mind, body, and spirit goals that will help you focus on God and work through the process of reconciliation. We believe that part of this starts with taking care of the temple (the body) that God has given us for the Christ spark in us all. We are all different in shape and size and level of health, wellness, and physical capability, but we all have Christ within us. Therefore, we should take care of that temple that God has given us. A healthy body can do more for others and share the Christ love within us in whatever capacity we are called to serve. You are still called to serve, you still have a purpose, and God still has need for you even as you process your moral injury. We believe this journey is going to help bring you closer to God, to help you find purpose in what you've experienced, and hopefully find a way to use that experience to glorify Christ's kingdom.

Finally, within these pages are our thoughts, feelings, beliefs, and experiences with moral injury. We will use a lot of "I" statements since our experiences shaped our theological beliefs on the topics of trauma, health, wellness, and the path to reconciliation. If these thoughts and feelings and beliefs do not resonate with your own experience, that is okay. All of our experiences collectively are shaping the Christian community's testament to God in the world. It is all good when it is done for the love of Christ. We hope that these meditations help you along on your journey and that you feel free to make them your own so they work within your own set of thoughts, feelings, beliefs, and experiences. Through strong minds, strong bodies, and strong spirits, we can walk with Christ all the days of our lives. Join us over the next forty days on your personal *Christ Walk Crushed* experience and see yourself transformed.

THOUGHTS TO PONDER

1. What is my goal?

_____

_____

_____

2. How do I feel about my goal? Is it reasonable/attainable/realistic? If not, how can I make it something that I will stick with for the next forty days?

_____

_____

_____

3. Who can I reach to help me out on my journey?

_____

_____

_____

My physical goal for *Christ Walk Crushed* the next forty days is:

_____

_____

_____

My spiritual goal for *Christ Walk Crushed* the next forty days is:

_____

_____

_____

My mental goal for *Christ Walk Crushed* the next forty days is:

_____

_____

_____

*And Moses swore on that day, saying, "Surely the land on which your foot has trodden shall be an inheritance for you and your children forever, because you have wholeheartedly followed the Lord my God." —*Joshua 14: 9

DAY 1 What Is Contrition?

BIBLICAL BIG IDEA #1

The LORD is near to the brokenhearted, and saves the crushed in spirit. —Psalm 34:18

Me: Hey God?
God: Yes?
Me: This world blows.
God: I know. That's why you need Jesus.

I do most of my running and walking on the ten-mile gravel trail that rings Lady Bird Lake. Since many of my runs are in the dark, I have to pay close attention to the ground, so I don't make an unexpected fall and embed some of the pea gravel in my knee. Unlike smooth river stones, gravel has sharp edges because of how it's made.

Gravel is made by turning big rocks into little rocks. Large rocks are crushed with machines until they're the size of a pea. It's a noisy process and it creates sharp edges. When life events crush us, it's often a noisy process and creates sharp edges. The noise drowns out the normal channels of communication with God, with others, and with our own sense of self. When it's over, we find that we are smaller, with many sharp edges. Life-crushing events have a way of changing our identity, causing disorientation and confusion. Like crushed gravel, we find ourselves trodden under the feet of others who do not know what they do.

The word "contrition" simply means "crushed." Whatever solid state we were in before our traumatic event, we are no longer in that state. We are smaller—broken and ground down by the gears and grinders of life. We are crushed.

Contrition is being aware of how much we are crushed by our own failures or the failures of others. This is a very risky place to be in. When I came home from the Iraq war to a broken marriage, I felt crushed by what happened to me. I felt like I no longer recognized who

I was. I also knew that, like crushed gravel, I had some sharp edges. I was edgy, and found it hard to enjoy anything, even my two wonderful children. I lashed out at people who cared about me and self-destructed with alcohol. I felt disconnected from other people, from myself, and especially from God.

It's taken me a long time to realize that just at the moment when I felt farthest from God because I was crushed, I was actually closer to God than I had ever been before. "The LORD is near to the brokenhearted, and saves the crushed in spirit," the psalmist writes. Being crushed brings God near. Being crushed in spirit brings salvation.

THOUGHTS TO PONDER

1. Was there an event in your life, large or small, that crushed you?

_____

_____

_____

2. Where was God when this happened to you? (There are no wrong answers, just go with your gut reaction.)

_____

_____

_____

3. What was the worst thing about the event that you've never told anyone about?

_____

_____

_____

DAY 1   Steps taken: _____   Miles journeyed: _____

Exercise chosen: _____

Something I thought about: _____

_____

_____

_____

_____

Something I need to pray about: _____

_____

_____

_____

_____

What Separates Us from God?

BIBLICAL BIG IDEA #2

For perverse thoughts separate people from God, and when his power is tested, it exposes the foolish; because wisdom will not enter a deceitful soul, or dwell in a body enslaved to sin. —Wisdom 1:3–4 (RSV)

Me: Hey God?

God: Yes?

Me: Why do I keep doing the same thing over and over and expecting things to be different?

God: Because it's the nature of humans to think they've got it all figured out.

As you walk on today's journey, I want you to think about Sin. We'll be talking about sin for a couple of chapters because it's important. All humans sin. Even prolific Christian writers. In fact, we may be more in touch with or aware of our sins because we write. I am a passionate person. I love fiercely, but I am also quick to anger. Frustration can simmer beneath my exterior when I think things aren't going my way. In fact, my children were recently describing my work and said, "Mommy writes about health policy. She gets mad when people don't listen to her." I cringed. Reacting with anger isn't what God teaches us. These sort of behaviors (and others) separate us from God. Most of the time we don't think about how our behaviors disconnect us from God. Perhaps we sin because we try to figure things out on our own. Humans are generally fallible; we screw up a lot of times, even when we are trying not to. This does not mean we are bad people, it just means we are a broken lot that needs the grace of God to figure out how to get back on track.

All of us sin. Just because we love God deeply doesn't mean that we haven't sinned. (If you've read any of our other books, you would know that we've both sinned quite a bit.) In both of our traumatic experiences, David and I tried to figure things out on our own. We went through stages of anger at God, rebellion against God, grief and loneliness as we wondered if God could ever forgive us our sins. And we experienced joy as we came to realize that God is ever faithful even when we are sinful creatures.

So, what is sin? Sin is any action that separates us from the love of God. The actions that separate us from God are unloving actions. Jesus came to teach us God loves us and had given the Law (such as the Ten Commandments) to help us avoid those kinds of unloving actions. We tend to think of sin as those things we only do to others, but we can also have unloving thoughts of ourselves and harmful actions directed to our own bodies. When we go through a traumatic event, there is a component of self-loathing that causes us to sin against ourselves.

When I was diagnosed with cancer, I blamed myself. I felt unworthy of God's love. I felt completely betrayed and left by God. I was a good girl. I am and was a God-fearing, Jesus-loving, trying-hard-to-practice-my-Christian faith gal. I often thought (wrongly) that all those good behaviors were going to protect me from bad things happening my life. I thought I had a "Get Out of Jail Free" card tucked in my back pocket. I was doing everything so right, how could things go wrong?

But they do. And they did. And things will probably get upended again before I die. The world has a way of throwing things at you. Just because you are going through something bad now doesn't mean that it won't ever happen again. That's why finding your way back to God is so important.

Jesus died to take our sins upon himself. He showed us *how* we should live for one another and how to love one another: selflessly. God realizes that we are flawed, and we continue to sin, but the gift of Jesus' love and crucifixion gives us hope that we can aspire to love as much as God loves us. A just and perfect God could not simply sweep sin under the carpet and go on running a perfect universe, allowing us to get away with murder (literally and figuratively). The gift of Jesus' life gave *us* the promise of life everlasting with God if we follow in the way of Christ. God's grace doesn't mean that sin doesn't happen, it means we have a vision of the way things are supposed to be when the bad things do happen, which involves turning back to God in Jesus.

The first step begins when we identify what is making us feel separated from God. From there, we can work on the steps needed to find our way back. That process of the journey will help us explore love and help us to know that we are very much loved, forgiven, and that there's a place for us in this crazy journey of life. As you walk today, think about how you have sinned against God.

THOUGHTS TO PONDER

1. Do you feel separated from God?

_____

_____

_____

2. What do you think has separated you from God?

_____

_____

_____

3. Why do you feel it has separated you from God?

_____

_____

_____

DAY 2 Steps taken: _____ Miles journeyed: _____

Exercise chosen: _____

Something I thought about: _____

_____

_____

_____

_____

Something I need to pray about: _____

_____

_____

_____

_____

What Is Remorse?

BIBLICAL BIG IDEA #3
All of them moaning over their iniquity.
All hands shall grow feeble,
all knees turn to water.
They shall put on sackcloth,
horror shall cover them.
Shame shall be on all faces. —Ezekiel 7:16b–18a

Me: Hey God?
God: Yes?
Me: Why are you looking at me like that?
God: Wait, what? I wasn't looking at you.

"I shouldn't have drunk so much last night," I said to my running buddy, as we met at zero dark thirty at the parking lot. I continued, "I feel awful." Whether it's too much to drink or too much to eat, I often have remorse during many a morning workout. "Buyer's remorse" happens often in a consumerist culture. We've all bought things we know we don't need or really want.

Remorse is an emotion we feel when we miss the mark or break the moral code we keep inside us, at least until the moment we break it. Because moral codes come from so many sources, we usually need to sort out with a therapist or spiritual director whether we are feeling shame or guilt. Sociologist Brené Brown's excellent research work[1] makes the distinction between shame and guilt this way: Guilt says, "I made a mistake," Shame says, "I am a mistake." The good news is that we are not mistakes, even though we make mistakes.

Shame leads to self-destruction; guilt can lead to a new life, a new start, and a new joy. No matter how bad we feel the morning after, we

---

1. https://brenebrown.com

must remember that God loves us truly and deeply. God does not see us as mistakes, even when we make mistakes. Truly, as the prayer that opens the Ash Wednesday service says, "Almighty and everlasting God, you hate nothing you have made."[2]

Our feelings of remorse are powerful and painful, and they can paralyze us. This is a very critical moment in our journey to healing. This is where we are most tempted to despair, self-destruct and stop dead in our tracks. It is possible to be dead while still alive, the real walking dead. You can see why ancient people wore sackcloth in times of remorse and repentance. They wanted their outward appearance to reflect how they felt inside.

In spite of the risks, this critical moment of our journey holds within it huge possibilities. During a 100-mile race my pacer shared a story with me during the hours of 10:00 p.m. to midnight. He told me how he grew up in church then left it. He was sitting on his couch one night after a very painful breakup, smoking weed and drinking. He was feeling awful about himself and how he always seemed to end up in the same predicament, on the same couch. He was feeling remorse. It was in that moment when he heard God speak to him. God told him to get up and go to church the next day. He did, and to make a long story short, that encounter brought him back into a community of love and hope. He went from poor health to running 100-milers, and from serial breakups to a healthy marriage.

THOUGHTS TO PONDER

1. What event prompted you to feel remorse?

---

2. Book of Common Prayer, 264.

2. What did you do when you felt remorse?

_____

_____

_____

3. Have you been able to see the difference between shame and guilt in your own story?

_____

_____

_____

DAY 3 Steps taken: _____   Miles journeyed: _____

Exercise chosen: _____

Something I thought about: _____

_____

_____

_____

Something I need to pray about: _____

_____

_____

_____

_____

4 What Is Penitence?

BIBLICAL BIG IDEA #4

Do not rejoice over me, O my enemy;
when I fall, I shall rise;
when I sit in darkness,
the LORD will be a light to me. —Micah 7:8

Me: Hey God?

God: Yes?

Me: I am so sorry. Sorrysorrysorrysorrysorry. . . I say this a lot.
I'm sorry.

God: I know. It's okay. I love you anyway.

Penitence is the act of expressing remorse, grief, and sorrow over what separates us from God. In our current pop-culture-filled world, we tend to have flashbacks to *The Da Vinci Code* when we think of penance for our sins where the monk is self-flagellating himself with the cat-o'-nine-tails; a bloody affair. People equate penitence with beating themselves up, but we don't need to in order to recognize that we are sorry for the things that we have done or left undone. Like many things with our faith and spiritual practices, true penitence is the outward signs of those things we've inwardly digested and come to terms with about ourselves. Unfortunately, we often exhibit behaviors that we think express penitence through mental, physical, and spiritual self-flagellation, but we haven't truly inwardly digested and accepted that no matter what we do, God forgives us if we are truly and sincerely repentant.

Self-abuse is not the same thing as being penitent.

I can be sorrowful and remorseful about those things that separate me from God and still continue to do those things that separate me from God, digging into an even deeper hole. I am very good at repeating the same thing over and over while expecting things to be different. Like every step on a journey, we first have to acknowledge those things that separate us from God (awareness), express a true inward desire to change things from the way they are to a new vision of togetherness with God (penitence), and then we need to take action. Penitence is not just expressing the sorrow, it's the outward expression that we want things to be different. We want to be together with God again. We are acknowledging that something is not quite right with our own personal *feng shui*. We might not quite yet believe that everything can be made right or that we are worthy of that forgiveness. Perhaps we still blame ourselves for what happened in our lives. The steps towards penitence acknowledge that things are off kilter and that things need to be different if we are going to survive.

I knew about nine months into my cancer diagnosis that things weren't okay in my spiritual and mental world. I was doing great (more or less) coping with the physical things that were going on, but I had been so intent on trying to defeat this cancer thing on my own, I left God somewhere behind me. In addition, with all the gung-ho attitude of be-all, do-all, I never really addressed how super pissed off at God I was for giving me cancer in the first place. (Not that God gave me cancer, but I sure did want a Gandalf-like wizard waving a magic wand to make it all go away.) I never acknowledged how I was trying to literally run away from my diagnosis on my runs, or how my once-healthy behaviors turned to not-so-healthy ones in a subconscious effort to punish myself for whatever I did wrong to get cancer. I was going, going, going in the immediacy of dealing with a traumatic diagnosis so that all of a sudden, I ended up in a deep hole wondering, "Where is God?"

A sure sign that things are off balance on your mind, body, or spiritual journey: your body hurts, you are mentally exhausted all the time, you pretty much hate anything to do with the church and God, and you are miserable. Dejected as a person, friend, lover, spouse, child, and/ or parent. These are all signs that somehow you've taken a step off the path *with* God and are walking a dark road by yourself. Some people will be aware that they are separated from God and need help. Others will need a buddy to tell them they need to get back on the right path.

When we come to the realization we've become separated from God we grieve. I think our bodies know that we need to be right and tight with our maker. Our soul craves for the balance that a life with God brings. Acknowledge the grief and sorrow that you are (or have been) separated from God and you need to find your way back. That's what *Christ Walk Crushed* is all about.

THOUGHTS TO PONDER

1. Are you grieving?

_____

_____

_____

2. What does your journey look like right now? Are you on a path that you want to stay on?

_____

_____

_____

3. What are some things you've done to beat yourself up about events in life?

_____

_____

_____

4. Have these actions done anything to make you feel closer to God or further away?

_____

_____

_____

DAY 4   Steps taken: _____   Miles journeyed: _____

Exercise chosen: _____

Something I thought about: _____

_____

_____

_____

_____

Something I need to pray about: _____

_____

_____

_____

_____

5 What Has Been Done and Left Undone?

BIBLICAL BIG IDEA #5

"What do you think? A man had two sons; he went to the first and said, 'Son, go and work in the vineyard today.' He answered, 'I will not'; but later he changed his mind and went. The father went to the second and said the same; and he answered, 'I go, sir'; but he did not go. Which of the two did the will of his father?" They said, "The first." Jesus said to them, "Truly I tell you, the tax collectors and the prostitutes are going into the kingdom of God ahead of you. For John came to you in the way of righteousness and you did not believe him, but the tax collectors and the prostitutes believed him; and even after you saw it, you did not change your minds and believe him. —Matthew 21:28–32

Me: Hey God?
God: Yes?
Me: Yes, yes is my answer. I'll do it.
God: Ok, I'll believe it when I see it.

During my time in the Marine Corps, I was on the receiving end of numerous orders. Being told what to do, often in a loud voice by a scary sergeant, is a hallmark of military service. Being able to follow orders while all hell is unleashed is a necessary skill for a soldier to have.

Disobeying orders in the military is illegal and often results in serious prosecution and punishment. Like sergeants, parents give orders too, and every family is different. Every parent has different expectations about what orders are acceptable to obey or disobey. "Because I said so," has ended many well-reasoned arguments.

The story Jesus told about these two sons is so ordinary—who hasn't said, "Yes, I'll go!" then rolled their eyes when dad left the room? The point Jesus is making here with this relatable story is that it doesn't matter what we say, it matters what we do.

Søren Kierkegaard, a nineteenth-century Danish writer, said the son who said "Yes" got immediate applause. Everybody loves a "Yes." Meanwhile, the son who said, "No" was instantly booed. However, after some time went by, the loud applause for the "Yes" son faded, and nothing happened. In fact, Kierkegaard states we often have to say "No" before we can say "Yes" to God's call to us.

When I came home from Iraq I felt very isolated from other people. I had been a "Yes Man" my whole life, always trying to get people to like me, always seeking their applause. But now, as my world began to shrink, I found myself saying "No." I said "No" to God, which, at first, was disturbing to me and many who witnessed it. But, looking back, I can say that "No" was the first honest thing I had ever said to God. It was as if I needed to say it. Looking back, I couldn't write this today if I hadn't said "No" at least once.

THOUGHTS TO PONDER

1. Have you ever said "Yes" to God, then not done anything?

_____

_____

_____

2. Have you ever said "No" to God, then went ahead and did the good thing you knew was right?

_____

_____

_____

DAY 5 Steps taken: _____ Miles journeyed: _____

Exercise chosen: _____

Something I thought about: _____

_____

_____

_____

_____

Something I need to pray about: _____

_____

_____

_____

_____

6 What Are God's Laws?

BIBLICAL BIG IDEA #6

The rest of the people, the priests, the Levites, the gatekeepers, the singers, the temple servants, and all who have separated themselves from the peoples of the lands to adhere to the law of God, their wives, their sons, their daughters, all who have knowledge and understanding, join with their kin, their nobles, and enter into a curse and an oath to walk in God's law, which was given by Moses the servant of God, and to observe and do all the commandments of the Lord our Lord and his ordinances and his statutes.
—Nehemiah 10:28–29

Me: Hey God?
God: Yes?
Me: What happens when I break your laws?
God: You repent.

God gave us a basic set of rules to follow for a couple of reasons. One, people like rules. Rules make it more-or-less clear how we are supposed to act as humans. Have you ever wondered what the world would be like if we simply followed God's most important law?

You shall love the Lord your God with all your heart, and with all your soul, and with all your mind. You shall love your neighbor as yourself. —Matthew 22:37, 39

The world would be a lot better place if we focused on these two commandments and stopped wasting time over everything else. God also knows we need these rules because we screw up all the time. It's *hard* to love your neighbor as yourself because we want to justify that love, using a measuring stick on someone else's behavior to see if they really deserve the love we are supposed to give them. We also "one-up" each other on our behavior sticks and feel self-righteous about our own habits compared to others. This creates a vicious cycle justifying our behaviors in our eyes, not God's.

This doesn't fly in God's eyes. God's love isn't given based on our behavior. We freely get that love by grace. The murderer down the street gets just as much of God's love as I do even though I've never killed anyone. While we may want to argue this idea, it's also *great* that God is so awesome to seek out each of us as our own person, worthy of God's love, just 'cause. Do you know why? This kind of love paves the way for our redemption and forgiveness. No matter what's happened to you, no matter what you've done, no matter the trauma and pain in your life, you can still be forgiven.

God does expect us to walk in love with one another. That's where God's rules come in to play. People like to argue about the efficacy of God's laws, but really, if we are following the golden rule, the rest kind of hang on the two big ones. If we love God and love our neighbor it makes it really hard to justify lying, adultery, thievery, murder, jealousy, greed, and so on. While many may want to hang the commandments out with the laundry, the truth is if you really love God and love your neighbor, none of those rules should be deal breakers in our relationship with God.

However, we are human. As a result, we screw up ALL. THE. TIME. with these rules. They are *hard*! Some are harder than others while some are easier. But God expects the best of each of us since we are made in God's image. That means when we do screw up, fail, break the rules, majorly dis the commandments, THEN we need to do something about it. When this happens, God asks us to repent, calling us back every day, every time. To be in communion with God means we need to recognize those things that break our relationship with God. So, we need to recognize those things that separate us from God and do something about it. God wants you. You are so very important to God. God would not have made you without reason. Sometimes when we drift in a sea of loneliness, regret, grief, pain, self-loathing, it's really hard to believe that we are loved. David and I are here to tell you that it's true; we've both swum in that sea and know the pain. We both know what it's like to break the rules and what it's like to crawl back to God with a firm realization that we are really nothing without the love of God.

THOUGHTS TO PONDER

1. Are you sinking or swimming?

_____

_____

_____

2. What sort of behaviors are you currently demonstrating that may be separating you from God?

_____

_____

_____

3. How do you need to repent?

_____

_____

_____

DAY 6 Steps taken: _____ Miles journeyed: _____

Exercise chosen: _____

Something I thought about: _____

_____

_____

_____

Something I need to pray about: _____

_____

_____

_____

_____

What Is Sin?

BIBLICAL BIG IDEA #7

Happy are those whose transgression is forgiven,
  whose sin is covered.
Happy are those to whom the LORD imputes no iniquity,
  and in whose spirit, there is no deceit.
While I kept silence, my body wasted away
  through my groaning all day long.
For day and night your hand was heavy upon me;
  my strength was dried up as by the heat of summer.
Then I acknowledged my sin to you,
  and I did not hide my iniquity;
I said, "I will confess my transgressions to the LORD,"
  and you forgave the guilt of my sin. —Psalm 32:1–5

Me: Hey God?
God: Yes?
Me: Everything hurts?
God: Everything always does.

On today's journey I hope you can start to make a connection between your spiritual life and your physical life. We live in a world that makes a sharp split between the spiritual and the physical, and for some good reasons. After all, we don't want to live in a world where our oncologist simply tells us we coveted our neighbor's Jeep too many times and that's the cause of disease. No, there isn't always a cause and effect between the spiritual and the physical, but we should not be so quick to burn the bridge between the two.

Exploring the link between our spiritual lives and our physical experiences is a constant theme in our Holy Scripture. Psalm 32 describes how our refusal to acknowledge our faults, our lack of forgiveness, and our denial can cause our bodies to "waste away." We groan and cannot sleep, even as we find ourselves exhausted. I know what this feels like all too well.

After my experience of war and divorce, I was very angry. I was angry at myself and at others who I felt had betrayed me. My anger drove me to intense running and exercising, which made me seem very healthy. But no one could see how much pain I was in. I had aches, pains, and frequent illnesses that felt like the flu but were un-diagnosable. I truly know what the psalmist is describing, I felt it.

Having physical manifestations of spiritual disease doesn't make us "crazy," it just makes us human. Go to the doctor when you're sick. Tell the doctor about what is going on in your personal life, work life, and family life. Find a spiritual counselor or sage to share your story with, too. This is a journey that takes time, so take your time.

THOUGHTS TO PONDER

1. During a time of extended illness or pain, have you ever noticed any spiritual changes in your life?

_____

_____

_____

2. List the names of three people you could tell about your spiritual and physical aches and pains.

_____

_____

_____

DAY 7   Steps taken: _____   Miles journeyed: _____

Exercise chosen: _____

Something I thought about: _____

_____

_____

_____

_____

Something I need to pray about: _____

_____

_____

_____

_____

How Do We Feel When Separated from God?

BIBLICAL BIG IDEA #8

But where are your gods
that you made for yourself?
Let them come, if they can save you,
in your time of trouble;
for you have as many gods
as you have towns, O Judah. —Jeremiah 2:28

Me: Hey God?
God: Yes?
Me: Where are you?
God: Here.

Let's delve into sin a bit further. Where is the distance in your life from God and why is it there? Sometimes those things that separate us from God are obvious, such as when we are cruel to others, when we lie, steal, covet, cheat, murder. Some behaviors are more insidious: self-centeredness, drug and alcohol abuse, arrogance, vanity, gluttony, and others are more subtle things that separate us from God. The quiet sins are those things we think we can get away with. Those are the "hidden" sins we try to justify as not really sins, because they don't really hurt anyone else, they only hurt ourselves. Sins—things that separate us from God—come in all sorts of shapes, sizes, vices, and negligent behaviors. Even those within ourselves and pointed towards ourselves. We can hurt ourselves as much as we hurt others with our sins.

One of my sins is arrogance. I think I can do most things without God. I often think I know better than God. This arrogance has led me to lie to myself as well as others time and time again. This behavior makes me think about myself. All. The. Time. . . and not about God, others, or where my attention should be. I am very good at making things about me—not God. When I got cancer, after the initial shock and pain wore off, my attitude was: "I've got this. Thanks, God, you can go now. I'm back in charge." It was such a lie. I was the biggest faker of how well I was doing, using all sorts of behaviors to justify everything because I had cancer. I'd punish my body with exercise, telling myself I was being "healthy" ; eat all the junk food—because you know, I have cancer, my good diet evidently didn't matter before, why worry about it now; have one extra drink or another because, hey, I have cancer. . . and so on and so forth, because you know, I have cancer, anything goes. I was secretly and horridly angry with God, angry with myself, and angry at the world for my having cancer. I could fake it on the outside with the best of them, but on the inside I was a lonely, miserable mess, convinced I was being punished for something. These spirals of negative thoughts will drown you and pull you deeper into the abyss of self-loathing. When you're adrift in that sea of awful, you think you are swimming, but really you are sinking.

Separated from God by my thoughts, feelings, and actions, I felt ill. I knew things were off. My body ached, and not just from disease. My heart was wounded. I would look in a mirror and the reflection I would see was a shattered form of me that no one else could see. But I could, wondering if I would ever be pieced back together again, feeling fragile and weak. I had no interest in people. I was lethargic. The things I used to enjoy brought me little happiness. It became harder and harder to find things that brought a genuine smile to my face. I felt discombobulated, like I was going through the motions. I didn't feel like me as I remembered me.

Does any of this resonate? A lot of what I describe is a classic description of depression: the feeling that you can't keep your head above water, so why bother. Sometimes it seems like it would be so much easier to just slip beneath the waves. It wouldn't, but it feels that way. That's when we have to recognize that our feelings are driving and manipulating our thoughts and our perceptions about reality. Depression often goes hand in hand with the "crushed" experience. When you've gone through hell and back, events in your life seem to be out of control, or everything you thought you understood was ripped out from under you, at some point in your experience you'll feel depressed. It's an oh-so-normal, but not-normal response to s-*%# happening. And it can take over your life. It sucks big-time. Depression blows.

There are physical and mental manifestations to depression. It can be a gateway to other things: drug and alcohol abuse, self-harm, suicide, hurting others, broken relationships, and more. I say this not to make you feel bad about being depressed—it's normal to become depressed after a traumatic event—but it's not so good to do nothing about it. Depression can be life-threatening; everyone should take it seriously and get help. I know I did. Depression runs in my family and framed my entire childhood as my dad struggled with his demons. I knew this wasn't something I could blow off.

I had to get back. I needed to do something. Desperately, I began to realize I was nothing without God. I cannot live my life, live with cancer, raise my kids, and do the things I want to do without God. God was a lifeline for me during the acceptance phase of my reconciliation process. When tragedy comes knocking, it is difficult to find meaning, understanding, or purpose in the event without God. Life happens, and with God we have the promise that whatever happens, it isn't the end of the story. There is so much more for us. When we repent and keep our covenant with God we have that promise of more to come. There is something more that comes from these events that shape us, these events that seem like random occurrences. God doesn't let these things happen, but God tells us that amazing things will happen when grace is mixed into the mess of our lives. God has promised us that through the resurrection of Christ all will be made right again one day. It might not be today, but one day, there is a promise that all will be right.

On today's journey think about how you feel and how that might be separating you from God.

THOUGHTS TO PONDER

1. On a scale of 1–10, how depressed do you feel?

_____

_____

_____

2. Do you have a friend, battle buddy, priest, therapist, family member you can talk to about your feelings?

_____

_____

_____

3. Are you wondering, "Where is God?"

_____

_____

_____

DAY 8   Steps taken: _____   Miles journeyed: _____

Exercise chosen: _____

Something I thought about: _____

_____

_____

_____

_____

Something I need to pray about: _____

_____

_____

_____

_____

What Is the Impact of Our Sin?

BIBLICAL BIG IDEA #9

The LORD struck the child that Uriah's wife bore to David, and it became very ill. —2 Samuel 12:15

Me: Hey God?
God: Yes?
Me: Who did I hurt?
God: More of us than you'll ever know.

Of all the stories of sin in the Bible, none rivals the saga of David and Bathsheba. The story is so compelling, so universal, it is as much at home in 1000 BCE as it is today. Most of us can relate to every character in it at one time or another in our lives, which is sad, but true. If you don't know the story, read it now in 2 Samuel 11–12, or listen to Leonard Cohen's song "Hallelujah"[3] a couple of times.

In 1951, Gregory Peck played King David in the lavish film *David and Bathsheba*. Before Nathan the Prophet confronts the adulterous and murderous king, David sees flashbacks of when he killed the Philistine giant Goliath in one-on-one combat and other victories over the Philistines. It is as if the director wants the viewer to know that everything is connected: Goliath, David's victories, and the blood that still clings to David's hands. Nathan confronts his king with a short story that concludes with, "You are the man." David is struck with conviction, and in the coming days, the child of his adulterous union dies a lingering death. The death of David's son begins a series of deaths, betrayals, and plagues that break David's power and prestige. The most

---

3. https://www.youtube.com/watch?v=YrLk4vdY28Q (accessed September 16, 2018).

tragic, in my mind, is the betrayal by his own son Absalom. It is as if the sins David committed were like a stone thrown into a calm pond, with ripple effects that keep on hitting the shore.

It is clear from reading King David's story, or seeing the Gregory Peck film (or even the epic 1985 "King David" starring Richard Gere) that all of David's life is connected. David's early traumas, his losses, and his betrayals all play into the deadly events of that spring and the days that followed. All of our sin was a bitter cocktail mixed long ago by evil done to us by people who had evil done to them. And it doesn't stop with us. Our sin ripples to our children, our neighbors, our coworkers, and some whom we will never meet.

How do I know this? I know this because I did it. After Iraq and my divorce, I wanted to feel powerful, so I entered relationships with women I could quickly end. I felt like the wrongs done to me in Iraq and my first marriage gave me a free pass to ignore the feelings of others. I know I hurt people during this time with my dishonesty, my arrogance, and my inability to think about anyone but myself.

So much of my healing journey has been making an honest assessment of the people I hurt, including my ex-wife, who I have always felt hurt me way more than I hurt her. In the convulsions of emotional pain, we often miscalculate how balanced the scales are. On a running pilgrimage from Springfield, Illinois, to Washington, DC, so many of these memories came back to me—memories of the ways I had hurt other people. In the solitude of the open road, with no phone or friends, I couldn't escape the long-buried memories of who I hurt. I needed to face these realities, and they started what I can now see as a journey toward healing.

Perhaps you need to go on this journey, so I challenge you today to walk without headphones or phone. Listen to your heart, and the spirit within you. You will know the truth, and the truth will set you free.

THOUGHTS TO PONDER

1. List three people you think you might have hurt in your life.

_____

_____

_____

2. Write down the day or time period you hurt them.

_____

_____

_____

3. Consider how these events are related to other events of hurt and trauma in your life.

_____

_____

_____

DAY 9 Steps taken: _____ Miles journeyed: _____

Exercise chosen: _____

Something I thought about: _____

_____

_____

_____

_____

Something I need to pray about: _____

_____

_____

_____

_____

What Actions Are Taken during Contrition?

BIBLICAL BIG IDEA #10

The sacrifice acceptable to God
is a broken spirit;
a broken and contrite heart,
O God, you will not despise. —Psalm 51:17

Me: Hey God?

God: Yes?

Me: My spirit is broken. Bleeding. I am of no use.

God: I have use of everyone. The broken, the poor, the oppressed, the downtrodden. You all have purpose in my sight.

I confess to Almighty God, to his Church, and to you, that I have sinned by my own fault in thought, word, and deed, in things done and left undone; For these and all other sins which I cannot now remember, I am truly sorry. I pray God to have mercy on me. I firmly intend amendment of life, and I humbly beg forgiveness of God and his Church and ask you for counsel, direction, and absolution. —Book of Common Prayer, p. 447

As we've mentioned previously, through our own fault or the fault of circumstance, we have sinned. We have become separated and lost from God. We have recognized that separation and confessed our sins. We have acknowledged those things we have done and left undone. It can be quite freeing to name those things that we have done wrong. It can be liberating to ask forgiveness and not expect anything else in return. In the judgmental society in which we live, forgiveness is like gold. It is priceless, unexpected, and releasing. Forgiveness is like a great bowel movement. You feel ten pounds lighter.

More seriously, as we enter into the process of reconciliation, step one is acknowledging the sin in our lives. Step two is contrition.

37

Contrition is awesome. It's like the first step on a long race with the first mile done as you head toward the finish line—but there is still a long way to go. Contrition is demonstrating your action, purpose, and intent to change. A contrite heart seeks to move away from those behaviors that separate us from God and practice behaviors that draw us closer. Contrition is a state of being, a feeling in your heart and soul that acknowledges without God you are nothing. It's the acknowledgment that this entire process of healing is bigger than you and you cannot do it on your own.

When we seek behavior change, it can take six weeks for a habit to become a part of our regular daily lives. The experts say it takes six months or more of repetition for a behavior to become the norm for you. So, if you are practicing a behavior change to draw you closer to God, you have to do it over and over and over again for it to become a part of who you are.

When we have experienced a traumatic event sometimes the biggest behavior change is just showing up. Sometimes being present, acknowledging that something is off, and waiting for the answer and the guidance is the first thing we need. It's that first step of putting one foot in front of the other until we get comfortable with where we are going. The road to healing and coming back to God starts with one step (as cliché as that may sound) and even though it feels off and not quite right and not quite there, it's one foot in front of the other that gets us to the place where we want to be—making our behavior change a part of the norm and not the exception.

John the Baptizer wandered in the wilderness, the Israelites wandered the desert, and Jesus, too, wandered. I am sure they felt lost at times. They definitely experienced hunger. Perhaps, at times, they felt separated from God. But in each case, the wandering wasn't forever. There was more to the story. John came to prepare the way for Jesus. The Israelites became God's chosen people. Jesus resisted temptation. Each time, there was purpose to the wandering. At some point, the wandering will not be aimless, but rather driven by a purpose and goal. All of a sudden, you will realize, "Well duh! I'm here God! I get it! I hear, I see, I feel, I know! Send me God, send me!" And then you'll be shouting from the mountain top, not walking, but running because it feels so good to *feel* something and realize you are on the path back to

God. Keep putting one foot in front of the other. Your wanderings are not aimless. Each step takes you closer to where you want to be.

The burnt heart doesn't really know what feeling is until all of a sudden it starts beating a little faster, a little stronger. You *feel* the need to seek God. You *feel* the need to do whatever it takes to be back with God because it feels so good.

Contrition is all about showing up and taking that first step. On today's journey, think about taking this next step.

THOUGHTS TO PONDER

1. Did you show up today?

_____

_____

_____

2. Where did you show up?

_____

_____

_____

3. How did it feel?

_____

_____

_____

4. Where are you going to show up tomorrow?

_____

_____

_____

DAY 10   Steps taken: _____   Miles journeyed: _____

Exercise chosen: _____

Something I thought about: _____

_____

_____

_____

_____

Something I need to pray about: _____

_____

_____

_____

_____

DAY 11 What Is Confession?

BIBLICAL BIG IDEA #11

"If you forgive the sins of any, they are forgiven them; if you retain the sins of any, they are retained." —John 20:23

Me: Hey God?
God: Yes?
Me: I sinned.
God: I'm glad to hear you say that.

The word "confession," like the word "love," has a lot of meanings in the English language. In religious conversations you can confess your faith in the words of the Nicene Creed; in the courthouse the district attorney will read out a confession you wrote on the night you were arrested. The word used for confession in the Bible is *homologeo*, which is the combo of two words, "same" and "speak." Literally, the word translated "confession" means "to say the same as."

When we confess our faith, we are saying the same thing that God is saying about the way the plan of salvation works. When we confess our sins, we are saying what God is saying about what we have done and left undone. Confession is not an original creative work, it is simply acknowledging the way things really are.

Confession is painful. Confession requires us to say something about ourselves and how something is not right. Yesterday I made an appointment with my confessor, a priest who lives near me. I made the appointment because I remembered several situations I dealt with as an Army chaplain in Iraq. During my deployment, there were several members of my unit who sexually assaulted other members of my unit. The unit leadership investigated the allegations, I met with both the victims and the perpetrators, and then nothing happened. Well, at least it seems that way to me now. What happened was the victims and perpetrators were separated out to different companies (but stayed in the same larger unit—the battalion)—that was the solution. I would see the victims walking around, doing their jobs on deployment, and I would think they were just fine. But they weren't. From what I know about Military Sexual Trauma (MST) now, they were in a great deal of pain and distress. Yesterday I realized how I contributed to their pain and distress by my ignorance of what was really going on, as well as my trust in the system that shielded abusers. I was wrong. I failed them.

I'm glad the Army has changed the ways they now handle MST, but it doesn't change what happened during my deployment. It doesn't change how I failed these vulnerable, low-ranking soldiers. At this point, on Day 1 of my contrition, making an appointment to participate in "confession" (what is also known as the Sacrament of Reconciliation) is a must. Other forms of reconciliation may follow, but I know enough about myself to know I need to do this.

And so, tomorrow afternoon at 3:00 p.m. I'll meet with my confessor and will say what God says about my sin. I will say what I did during that deployment and I will say what I didn't do during that deployment. And then, my confessor will pray for me.

What my confessor and I will be doing can be traced back to the Bible verse above in John's gospel. Jesus is commissioning his disciples after his resurrection to share the good news with the world. He places on them his authority to forgive sins. It is comforting to know that two thousand years ago Jesus empowered my confessor to forgive my sin of not doing enough for the victims of sexual assault in my unit.

And it doesn't stop there. From that moment of forgiveness, I plan on going on a journey of forgiveness, which I will describe later. But the first step is to say, out loud, the same thing God says about what I did.

THOUGHTS TO PONDER

1. Have you ever asked someone to hear your confession?

_____

_____

_____

2. Who could you trust to hear something like that?

_____

_____

_____

DAY 11:   Steps taken: _____   Miles journeyed: _____

Exercise chosen: _____

Something I thought about: _____

_____

_____

_____

_____

Something I need to pray about: _____

_____

_____

_____

_____

12 How Do We Fail?

BIBLICAL BIG IDEA #12:

And the one who admits his fault will be kept from failure.
—Sirach 20:3

Me: Hey God?
God: Yes?
Me: I'm a failure.
God: No, you are a work in progress.

Think about ways you've failed as a Christian. Now, before you threaten anarchy on me about too much doom and gloom and essentially there's no hope (there's always hope—cue the *Star Wars* theme), I think it's important self-development to think of ways, actions, and places we can be more Christian in our everyday life. We fail horribly (well, maybe horribly is rather strong, but regularly) at being a Christian in our day-to-day lives and tend to save up those Christian behaviors for special occasions. We whip out Christianity like a magic wand and scatter those "Bless your hearts" with abandon while simultaneously failing to realize that God is calling us to act like God's people all the time.

Acting like a Christian is a part of the reconciliation process because we need to make a habit of putting God and God-like behaviors first in our lives. Our human nature is to be self-centered; however, Jesus continually asks us about others because he's trying to teach us that it's not all about you, or me, or ourselves. Our lives as Christians are to be devoted to others.

It is especially hard to live a life of intent, mindful, Christian behavior during the grieving period of a traumatic event because we get so wrapped up in the intense feelings of what we are experiencing. We start to believe there is no one else that could possibly understand what we are going through. We start to feel like an island. Heck, we start to feel like Pluto, abandoned in the far reaches of the solar system, neglected, rejected, renamed, relegated. Pluto gets it. The folly and capriciousness of humans can leave one with a serious case of identity crisis: Who are we? Where did we come from? What's the purpose of all this? Why the hell am I here?

Cue God. We should strive to follow Christ's example every day because it gives reason for our existence and purpose to the pain we feel from the trauma in our lives. God's grace, scattered daily, is far more powerful than the magical wand we whip out for special occasions. If we practice our faith daily and look outside of ourselves on a regular basis, we can begin to build a foundation of faith and trust that won't be crippled when we are interrupted by the ugly world around us.

A faith practiced daily builds wisdom and understanding that God doesn't promise us heaven on earth. God promises us, even in the midst of our gut-wrenching grief, that this is not the end of the story. The Christian hope is more than cancer, rape, murder, death, abuse, addiction, or whatever your pain because God's grace can be found through these experiences. If we allow it, these experiences—no matter how painful—can draw us deeper in relationship with God. The tribulations of the world seem to pale in comparison to a God that makes promises of steadfast love *despite* these things.

We fail to live as Christians every day. It's human nature and why God calls us to a life of discipline. It's why Jesus asks us to love one another—probably the hardest thing we can do. Sometimes grief and pain are so intense you hate yourself and maybe everyone else too. Practicing those Christian disciplines can help us to get over the hump of hate: prayer, worship, rest, and turn to Christ. See the old lady struggling to get the can off the shelf? Stop and help. Find a food pantry, soup kitchen, or homeless shelter and give one hour a week (more if you are able). See someone sitting alone? Buy them a coffee. Call your mother/father/sister/brother/friend and say hello. Say you are sorry out loud (even if there is no one there to listen). Thank God for one thing on a daily basis. Someone wants to cut you off in the road? Let them. Someone wants to cut ahead of you in the grocery line? Let them. Look around you for the little, everyday ways we can love another person.

When I was working myself out of my dark hole, I would go to the local food bank and stock the shelves. I would help families fill their bags of allotted food for the day and I would butcher my Spanish while trying to converse with those whose language is not English. People would ask me how I found time to do this on top of everything else going on. The secret is that this food bank was my lifeline. The food bank wasn't about me. It was about me realizing that there is a lot of suffering in the world and I wasn't the only hurting person out there. The food bank was about me finding love again and each day growing and nurturing that love. I have a special place in my heart for food banks and love to volunteer in them. These practices make me realize my mind, body, and spiritual health is more than taking a run and going to church. It makes me realize that this world is about more than me.

It's the practicing of an outward-facing habit, even if the feeling isn't there yet, that will help you on that journey back to yourself and back to God. These little acts help to grow love. And as love grows, healing follows. These are the ways we work (hard!) at being Christians on a daily basis. It takes practice to seek out something more than ourselves to gain a deeper relationship with God, which is where we will find the reconciliation and peace that we seek.

THOUGHTS TO PONDER

1. What was something you did today that wasn't about you?

_____

_____

_____

2. What was something you did (or didn't do) today in which you could have been a better Christian?

_____

_____

_____

3. Where were you looking for God? Did you find God? Why or why not?

_____

_____

_____

DAY 12: Steps taken: _____ Miles journeyed: _____

Exercise chosen: _____

Something I thought about: _____

_____

_____

_____

_____

Something I need to pray about: _____

_____

_____

_____

_____

How Does Trauma Separate Us from God?

BIBLICAL BIG IDEA #13

When it was evening on that day, the first day of the week, and the doors of the house where the disciples had met were locked for fear of the Jews. Jesus came and stood among them and said, "Peace be with you." —John 20:19

Me: Hey God?
God: Yes?
Me: I'm never going back there again. I'm never going anywhere again.
God: No worries. I'm coming to you.

Of all the stories of trauma from Iraq, I think it was the chow hall bombing that still haunts me. A chaplain friend of mine was eating with his soldiers in the chow hall when an insurgent ran into their midst wearing a vest full of bombs. The vest detonated, killing and wounding dozens of people. In an instant, a place that was thought to be a refuge from the deployment became a scene of carnage and crying. The blast not only shattered bodies and lives, it shattered everyone's illusion of safety.

I've heard Post Traumatic Stress Disorder (PTSD) described as the loss of the illusion of safety. Trauma, a Greek word for "wound," damages primarily our sense of safety—the sense we are okay. Trauma turns our world upside down, and changes everything we believe. For the disciples, the trauma of the trial, torture, and crucifixion of Jesus hurled them into a world of fear and hiding. John tells us they were behind locked doors, fearful they would be carted away to hang on crosses of their own.

Locking one's self away is a normal reaction to trauma, and many of us have done it after something goes terribly wrong. If God has given us a feeling of peace and safety before a trauma, this feeling about God is often shattered. Suddenly, we are alone. The God who we thought loved and protected us has disappeared, and all we can do is hide.

And it is precisely at this time, when we are hidden away behind locked doors, that God comes to us. Jesus comes to his disciples when they cannot come to him because of their trauma response.

After Iraq I felt like God abandoned me. I felt isolated from God and began to pull away from more and more people. It was at my lowest point I heard God speak to me. The message I heard one night was a message of overwhelming peace, that I was going to be okay. When I could not go to God, God came to me.

THOUGHTS TO PONDER

1. What illusion of safety was shattered in your trauma or loss?

_____

_____

_____

2. Where was God when you suffered a trauma or loss?

_____

_____

_____

3. What did you hear from God during that time?

_____

_____

_____

DAY 13: Steps taken: _____ Miles journeyed: _____

Exercise chosen: _____

Something I thought about: _____

_____

_____

_____

_____

Something I need to pray about: _____

_____

_____

_____

_____

Why Confess a Moral Injury?

BIBLICAL BIG IDEA #14

Anyone who maims another shall suffer the same injury in return. —Leviticus 24:19

Me: Hey God?

God: Yes?

Me: I've tried so hard to be good. Why did this happen? Why did you forsake me?

God: I have not forsaken you. I am faithful. The world's ways are not my ways and I am with you through it all.

We've described a sin as something that separates us from God. Often, our culture equates sin with something bad that someone does. This can be true, but it's not the only thing that separates us from God. Sometimes our thoughts and feelings as a result of events lead us to distance ourselves from God. This is a sin because it fails to account for God's grace that tells us all through the messiness of the Bible to "trust God!"

A moral injury is an insult to our psyche and soul by events and action of others over which we have little or no control. A moral injury shreds our understanding of the world and God as we know it and it prompts us to question, leave, become angry, disillusioned, practice risky behaviors, and so on. A moral injury is not always seen, but it produces emotional shame and is definitely felt by an individual. In many ways it is life- and personality-changing.

In the Bible God has shown us over and over again through the covenants established with people that "God's got this." When we fail to trust in God, even with our terrible moral injuries, we do sin. God understands our pain, grief, and wretchedness and forgives us anyway. God meets us in the middle of our suffering through Jesus; Jesus is fully

God and fully human to experience all of humanity's suffering. Thanks to the gift of the crucifixion and resurrection, God understands it all. God recognizes that the self-loathing and self-contempt that leads to our separation and sin is not the final way. We can also be brought back. Jesus was made fully whole in the resurrection: God's gift to us. This is reconciliation, being made whole though God.

I lost my hearing when I was twelve years old after being very sick for about three years. Later my dad had a psychotic break following a traumatic brain injury. Several years went by and my mom got cancer; then I got cancer. Throughout these years, I equated my faith with checking the boxes off a list of things I had to do for God to earn God's protection and forgiveness. I believed these bad things continued to happen to me because I wasn't good enough. There wasn't a litmus test I could pass because s-%$# was still going to happen. If you aren't aware, #badthingshappentogoodpeople.

Today I believe loss is simply a part of the human condition and no one gets through with a free pass. We will all experience something that causes us to pause, question, and hurt in response to events. It's in these moments that God is calling us to confess that, "Yes! This s%$# hurt my soul!" I'm aching, I'm lost, I'm alone, I am without God and I don't know how to find my way back. This is faith. Faith is dirty, ugly, and raw. Faith isn't a list. God is going to love me, forgive me, and welcome me no matter what I do (or did). I just need my heart to be focused on God.

From there you will seek the LORD your God, and you will find him if you search after him with all your heart and soul. —Deuteronomy 4:29

You shall love the LORD your God with all your heart, and with all your soul, and with all your might. —Deuteronomy 6:5

Remember the long way that the LORD your God has led you these forty years in the wilderness, in order to humble you, testing you to know what was in your heart, whether or not you would keep his commandments. —Deuteronomy 8:2

So now, O Israel, what does the LORD your God require of you? Only to fear the LORD your God, to walk in all his ways, to love him, to serve the LORD your God with all your heart and with all your soul. —Deuteronomy 10:12

Evidently, the Deuteronomist and I have something in common. We think a lot about what God requires. God requires my heart and soul. Only through God can my moral injury be healed, and it is through the process of confessing my injuries, just like a sin, that I have found my way back to communion with God. It's a wonderful, peaceful, easy feeling when you've found your way back and I am truly hopeful that each step of this journey is drawing you closer to that peaceful, easy feeling as well.

THOUGHTS TO PONDER

1. What is your moral injury?

_____

_____

_____

2. Can you confess it?

_____

_____

_____

3. How does it separate you from God?

_____

_____

_____

4. What's something you can do about that?

_____

_____

_____

DAY 14   Steps taken: _____   Miles journeyed: _____

Exercise chosen: _____

Something I thought about: _____

_____

_____

_____

_____

Something I need to pray about: _____

_____

_____

_____

_____

DAY 15 Why Is Confession Important?

BIBLICAL BIG IDEA #15

When they had finished breakfast, Jesus said to Simon Peter, "Simon son of John, do you love me more than these?" He said to him, "Yes, Lord; you know that I love you."
—John 21:15

Me: Hey God?
God: Yes?
Me: I can barely get my laundry folded and put away; how will I find time for confession?
God: It's your dirty laundry, no rush.

Finding time for the things we need to do is hard for many of us. It's hard for me, anyway. I seem to have energy for all kinds of activities, except for the ones that lead to a better life. At times I wonder if some of those old psychiatrists were right, that we subconsciously avoid things that cause pain.

Confession is a life or death matter, at least for me. The burden of moral injury, the burden of regret, the burden of things done and left undone are carried on our backs, visible to everyone but us. We can only distract ourselves for so long. Confession is one of the ways we lay those burdens down.

The story of Jesus' reconciliation with Peter after the resurrection starts with breakfast. I think that is always a good place to start. Just as we start each day with something to eat, or at least some bitter, black coffee, Peter starts his confession with breakfast. Many Christians down through the centuries have required confession before eating the bread and drinking from the cup at communion. This is a venerable practice, but it is not what happens here with Jesus and Peter. Peter desperately needs reconciliation after what he has done and left undone. He had denied with an oath that he knew Jesus, just when Jesus needed him most. Then he hid, ran away, and went back to fishing like nothing ever happened. But now, his teacher and friend are here with him, eating breakfast. It must have been an awkward meal, as I imagine it. But, there in the simple eating and drinking, something happens.

They eat first, a sign that they are already reconciled in some way. The confession and reconciliation that follows is a recognition of what has already happened when Jesus died on the cross and rose again. Confession is how we appropriate, realize, and digest what has already happened.

So, go and have breakfast first, then tell your story, and hear Jesus' words of love and healing that he speaks directly to you, "Peter, do you love me?" Yes, Jesus, we do love you.

THOUGHTS TO PONDER

1. What was the most awkward meal you've ever experienced?

_____

_____

_____

2. What is your answer to the question, "_____," do you love me?

_____

_____

_____

DAY 15 Steps taken: _____   Miles journeyed: _____

Exercise chosen: _____

Something I thought about: _____

_____

_____

_____

_____

Something I need to pray about: _____

_____

_____

_____

_____

Who Needs Confession?

BIBLICAL BIG IDEA #16

If we confess our sins, he who is faithful and just will forgive us our sins and cleanse us from all unrighteousness. —1 John 1:9

Me: Hey God?
God: Yes?
Me: I don't want to tell you what I did wrong.
God: What makes you think I don't know already?

In the Roman Catholic and Orthodox traditions, confession takes place with a priest as a conduit to the forgiveness of God. In the Episcopal and Anglican tradition, confession can take place in private or with a priest. In the Protestant traditions, confession is between you and God. No matter how it is done, all these traditions agree that confession is important. There is power in giving voice to those things you've done wrong (or not done) and in just asking for forgiveness. It's also fricking hard.

Confession is like having to own up to eating the last chocolate chip cookie when no one was looking. Or owning up to being less than you think you are. I'm not sure why, but just acknowledging you screwed up feels like you've been asked to storm the beaches of Normandy single-handedly. You don't really want to fess up because that might influence how the world perceives you. God forbid we look at each other in a new light. It ain't that hard and is something we shouldn't fear or dread because dang it, God *promises* us forgiveness. God already knows we are flawed. Only through the grace of God are we made whole. So why is it so hard? I don't know, but good things in life are often difficult. It doesn't mean we shouldn't do it.

Who should confess? Everyone should confess! Regardless of your faith tradition, confession is a good thing. It means getting stuff off your chest so you can move on. Confession moves us from the events of the past, into the present where grace is active and happening right now, so that we can look forward to the future with purpose and intent. A lot of times we look at confession only through the lens of mortal sins—those things that we do wrong, but as we noted previously, since moral injuries can separate us from God, it's important that we confess how those hurts, losses, injuries, and illnesses have also separated from God.

Verbalizing that you are hurt is a great way to move on. You cannot move on until you've acknowledged that something is separating you from where you want to be. Confessing your moral injury is a step in the right direction. It's admitting you are hurt and want to take the next steps toward healing and wholeness. It is always available, but it begins with you. If you aren't willing to acknowledge your hurt yet, it might be time to keep walking and come back when you are ready to move to the next step.

THOUGHTS TO PONDER

1. Have you ever practiced confession?

_____

_____

_____

2. What do you think of confessing to someone else? Does it make your skin crawl or fill you with hope? Either way, why?

_____

_____

_____

3. What do you need to confess?

_____

_____

_____

4. Are you ready to confess?

_____

_____

_____

DAY 16 Steps taken: _____ Miles journeyed: _____

Exercise chosen: _____

Something I thought about: _____

_____

_____

_____

_____

Something I need to pray about: _____

_____

_____

_____

_____

DAY 17 What Does Confession Do to the Body?

BIBLICAL BIG IDEA #17

But you made the nazirites drink wine,
* and commanded the prophets,*
* saying, "You shall not prophesy."*
So, I will press you down in your place,
* just as a cart presses down*
* when it is full of sheaves.*
—Amos 2:12–13

Me: Hey God?
God: Yes?
Me: My back hurts today.
God: Oh, let me take a look in that rucksack.

When the ghost of Jacob Marley appears to Ebenezer Scrooge in *A Christmas Carol*, he is completely decked out in heavy chains. Marley, a cruel miser, tells Scrooge he forged these chains in life by his greed. The association between sin and carrying burdens is an ancient one.

In the Scripture verses above, the prophet Amos speaks the words of God, who is angry at the people who forced the devout Nazirites to break their oath of abstinence and those who forbade the prophets from prophesying. For these two serious offenses, Amos says God will press down on these evil men, just as a heavily loaded cart presses down on itself. This is a vivid word picture of what happens when we sin. When we hurt other people, we incur a burden. We forge our own chains, we overload our own cart. And, if we take Amos's word for it, it seems that God is part of this somehow.

Our unconfessed sin is a burden to us, as well as a burden to those who love us. Often this load on our backs is visible to everyone but us. They try to help, but we have loaded our own rucksacks, we have overloaded our own carts, and we have forged our own chains. We know we're tired, but we often have a hard time figuring out why.

Confession lightens the load. It is the one way we can give these burdens to God, so God will carry them for us. As I think of Jesus, staggering under the weight of the cross on his way to Golgotha, I think of how he carried the weight of my sins, my burdens.

We carry these burdens in our bodies, for we are bodies. The soul/body distinction is nearly impossible to sort out for me, so I don't try. I know how much my back and neck hurt when I'm carrying something I need to confess. I know how physical that is.

When I am carrying a sack of sin on my back, I find it difficult to run. I seem sluggish, as all my energy is diverted from my legs to maintaining the load on my back. This is exhausting. When I am exhausted, I sometimes hear the words of Jesus in Matthew 11:28, "Come to me, all you that are weary and are carrying heavy burdens, and I will give you rest." Jesus wants to hear my confession. Jesus wants to give me rest. He loves us that much.

I speak from experience when I say confession will take a load off our bodies. Guilt and shame live in our bones and can be released through our mouths as we confess. We will feel better when more of our sin is given to God and our relationships with each other are on a path toward reconciliation. Then we can run and not be weary. Then we will walk and not faint.

THOUGHTS TO PONDER

1. Have you ever felt the physical burden of sin?

_____

_____

_____

2. Where in your body did you feel it?

_____

_____

_____

3. What are the physical activities you are unable to do when you feel the weight of contrition?

_____

_____

_____

DAY 17 Steps taken: _____   Miles journeyed: _____

Exercise chosen: _____

Something I thought about: _____

_____

_____

_____

_____

Something I need to pray about: _____

_____

_____

_____

_____

DAY 18 Are We Bad People to Need Confession?

BIBLICAL BIG IDEA #18

I prayed to the LORD my God and made confession, saying, "Ah, Lord, great and awesome God, keeping covenant and steadfast love with those who love you and keep your commandments." —Daniel 9:4

Me: Hey God?

God: Yes?

Me: I'm a bad person.

God: You aren't a bad person. You are made in my image. I am good; therefore, you are good. You sin, you stray, but like sheep that follow the good shepherd, you will always have a place with me.

On today's journey I want you to know that you are a good person. Whatever you are dealing with doesn't have to define you forever. It may impact you, mold you, mature you, and develop you, but the here-and-now pain doesn't have to be forever. It's easy to think that these things happen because we are bad people, and that having something to confess makes us immoral. It doesn't. You aren't an evil person for whatever happened to you. Just like I'm not an awful person because I lost my hearing, got cancer, and have a dad that's got a mental illness. David is not a lousy person because he suffers from post-traumatic stress disorder. Neither of us is a bad person because we tried to punish ourselves with harmful behaviors because of what we experienced. These things just happen. It's what we do with these challenges that defines us.

The practice of confession (it should happen more than once and should happen on a regular basis either with a clergy member or between you and God) gives us that opportunity to take our painful journey in a new direction. The practice of confession allows us to profess that we are less without God. The art of confession surrounds us with the comfort of grace in which we know that we are nothing without God. Confession equals nothing to something.

Like most things in life confession takes practice; a discipline that requires repetition to become the norm. If it feels awkward, it should. It takes time for it to become a part of who you are. It takes time and work to remind yourself that you are nothing without God. On your steps and journey, practice the confession with each step. Breathe each word into existence so that you express your admission with each step. Make the words of your declaration the steps you take on this part of your journey:

> *Have mercy on me, O God, according to your loving-kindness;*
> *in your great compassion blot out my offenses.*
> *Wash me through and through from my wickedness,*
> *and cleanse me from my sin.*
> *For I know my transgressions only too well,*
> *and my sin is ever before me.*
>
> *Holy God, Holy and Mighty, Holy Immortal One,*
> *have mercy upon us. Amen.* —Book of Common Prayer, 449

If this is too much all at once, break it down into a mantra you practice on your journey. Repeat in cadence and with each step:

> *Holy God, Holy Immortal One, have mercy upon us.*
> *Holy God, Holy Immortal One, have mercy upon us.*
> *Holy God, Holy Immortal One, have mercy upon us.*
> *Holy God, Holy Immortal One, have mercy upon us.*
> *Holy God, Holy Immortal One, have mercy upon us.*

Or this:

> *Have mercy on me, O God.*
> *Have mercy on me, O God.*
> *Have mercy on me, O God.*
> *Have mercy on me, O God.*
> *Have mercy on me, O God.*

Or this:

Pray for me, a sinner.
Pray for me, a sinner.
Pray for me, a sinner.
Pray for me, a sinner.
Pray for me, a sinner.

It doesn't have to be elaborate or complex to enter into the practice of confession. You are working on steps that draw you closer to God and not further away. Talking to God about what its wrong is one of those steps in the process. Regardless of being a "good" or "bad" person, we all have things that have happened that need to be confessed and addressed to draw us closer to God and not further away.

Pray for me. I, too, am a sinner. Amen.

THOUGHTS TO PONDER

1. Do you think you are a bad person? (circle one)

Yes   No   It's Complicated

2. Do you feel like you need to confess? (circle one)

Yes   No   It's Complicated

3. Why did you answer the way you did for either of these questions?

_____

_____

_____

4. What do you think of combining the spiritual practice of a confessing prayer with each step you take on your journey?

_____

_____

_____

DAY 18 Steps taken: _____ Miles journeyed: _____

Exercise chosen: _____

Something I thought about: _____

_____

_____

_____

_____

Something I need to pray about: _____

_____

_____

_____

_____

DAY 19 How Often Do We Confess?

BIBLICAL BIG IDEA #19:

For as the heavens are high above the earth,
so great is his steadfast love toward those who fear him;
as far as the east is from the west,
so far he removes our transgressions from us.
As a father has compassion for his children,
so the LORD has compassion for those who fear him.
For he knows how we were made;
he remembers that we are dust. —Psalm 103:11–14

Me: Hey God?
God: Yes?
Me: Oops, I did it again.
God: I've heard that song before.

Last night I attended a high school orchestra concert for my two oldest sons. Their school life has always been a mystery to me, ever since their mother and I divorced eleven years ago. So, these school events are always vivid reminders of how little I know of their weekday lives. After all, I've mainly seen them on the weekends for most of their lives. I get a little sad at these events, and so, as I congratulated my thirteen-year-old afterward and expressed my love for him and how I was proud of him, he said, "Dad, don't get all depressed." He knows me pretty well. So, I held back my tears, laughed, and was impressed by his quick-witted response to my feelings.

This morning I'm in a surgical center with my three-year-old son, who just had his tonsils removed. Needless to say, he is in pain, suffering as only a toddler can suffer.

The feelings I feel for my three children are overwhelming at times. Even as my wife and I held our toddler's extremely squirmy body in a vice grip so the nurse could squirt medicine into his mouth, I felt sad he was in so much pain, and that we had to be part of that pain. God's compassion for us is compared to this kind of love, a father's compassion for his children.

I am an imperfect father, quickly exasperated by these children who seem to be able to press every button I've ever had. But when I see them suffer, it breaks my heart. When my older boys struggle with relationships, with God, and with their own limitations, I cannot separate their struggles from my own. Is this what the psalmist is getting at? That God's compassion for us is so intense because God cannot separate God's self from us? If my relationship with my children is the metaphor for God's compassion for us, then it must be something like this.

And God's tenderness for us is expressed in how God removes our transgressions from us. Our wrongdoings are removed from us, as far as the east is from the west. This expression, "as far as the east is from the west," is an absurdity, a metaphor of infinity. If this is true, then there is an infinite number of times we can confess something, because there is infinite compassion in God's heart for us.

This is a fun message to preach and write, but it is very hard to believe—for ourselves and others. But this is why it's called faith; we must sometimes believe the possible-impossibles. And the most possible-impossible thing in the universe is that we have a second chance, that we have a third chance, and that we have a 333rd chance. Believing we are loved is so difficult when we are faced with reality, so we must contemplate how much a good parent loves their child. Perhaps that will give us some insight into how many times we can confess the same thing, over and over again.

THOUGHTS TO PONDER

1. Is love really love if it isn't infinite?

2. Where is the line God draws on how many times God will forgive?

_____

_____

_____

3. What would you do for your child, real or imaginary?

_____

_____

_____

DAY 19   Steps taken: _____   Miles journeyed: _____

Exercise chosen: _____

Something I thought about: _____

_____

_____

_____

_____

Something I need to pray about: _____

_____

_____

_____

_____

What Actions Do We Take during Confession?

BIBLICAL BIG IDEA #20

While Ezra was praying and making his confession, weeping and lying on the ground before the temple, there gathered around him a very great crowd of men and women and youths from Jerusalem; for there was great weeping among the multitude. —1 Esdras 8:91

Me: Hey God?

God: Yes?

Me: I am weeping and gnashing my teeth! I am beating my breast! I am pulling my hair! I lie down in agony!

God: Why?

Me: I'm trying to show contrition.

God: I can see your heart.

I am a bit of a dramatic person and have been known to weep, gnash my teeth, beat my breast, and fall down in agony. The psalmists are my spirit animals. I get the desire to make a big production. By God, if I am going to own up to my sins, it's going to be spectacular. Everybody is gonna know. God's not going to have any question that I'm owning up to my faults and deeds. I don't want any question about the way forward, so let's make it clear.

None of it matters, although the actions and drama often make us feel better. My crying is an outlet for the overwhelming emotion in my heart when dealing with my disease. The action makes me feel like I'm doing something, but at the end of the day, God already knows what's in my heart. God knows if I am trying to pull a fast one on confessing what's going wrong with me. God knows if I'm trying to slip an extra card into the playing deck. God knows where I am screwing up and knows when I am working towards making it right. God knows when we are in communion with one another and also knows when I am off trying to do my own thing (and usually failing).

If I recognize that God is all-knowing, all-seeing, in all times and all places, then I also must acknowledge that confession doesn't require any special actions from me. Confession is the truthfulness in my heart that God can see—no matter what. God knows when I'm faking it. God knows when you are faking it, too.

There aren't any elaborate genuflections, self-flagellations, or falling prostrate required. . . unless you want it. Christian traditions are an important part of what makes us a community of believers and some of these actions helps us on the road to recovery. You can cross yourself, do penance, use special language or words that come from you, give alms, and you can walk through doors backwards. You can do what works for you in confession, but at the end of the day, God is going to know what's in your heart.

> *For thus says the high and lofty one*
>   *who inhabits eternity, whose name is Holy:*
> *I dwell in the high and holy place,*
>   *and also with those who are contrite and humble in spirit,*
> *to revive the spirit of the humble,*
>   *and to revive the heart of the contrite.* —Isaiah 57:15

THOUGHTS TO PONDER

1. What actions do you like to express when you are confessing?

_____

_____

_____

2. How do they make you feel?

_____

_____

_____

3. What is God seeing in your heart right now?

_____

_____

_____

DAY 20   Steps taken: _____   Miles journeyed: _____

Exercise chosen: _____

Something I thought about: _____

_____

_____

_____

_____

Something I need to pray about: _____

_____

_____

_____

_____

What Is Satisfaction?

BIBLICAL BIG IDEA #21

Then Cain went away from the presence of the LORD, and settled in the land of Nod, east of Eden. —Genesis 4:16

Me: Hey God?

God: Yes?

Me: How do I forget this chapter of my life?

God: By remembering it really hard for the next couple of weeks.

Since this is a book, just pretend you hear the Rolling Stones singing about how they "Can't get no, satisfaction." In fact, I encourage you to pull the song up on YouTube right now.[4]

Ok, you've got it? Good.

Satisfaction is the part of reconciliation where the hard work happens. The church I belong to, the Episcopal Church, doesn't use this word that often, whereas the Roman Catholic Church does. For Roman Catholics, satisfaction has two parts: accepting the penance and penance. We'll cover penance tomorrow but accepting penance and doing penance are huge movements toward healing and hope.

We can see this pattern of accepting then doing penance in the story of Cain and Abel in Genesis 4. Cain, the first human child, is jealous of his brother, Abel, and kills him. When God comes to question him about the murder, Cain is sentenced to leave his community and wander, living the life of a fugitive. I'm always struck by how good God is at this whole thing, even though this is God's and humanity's first murder case!

God tells Cain he must wander the earth; Cain gets scared and says it's too difficult for him. After all, Cain is a farmer and farmers have to

---

4. https://www.youtube.com/watch?v=qAzqSYQ9X9U (accessed September 20, 2018).

stay in one place in order to plant and reap their crops. Because Cain complains, God relents and puts a mark of protection on Cain, so no one will kill him for committing fratricide, the murder of a brother.

Yes, I know this is God's first murder case, but God seems to know what God is doing. God doesn't kill Cain outright. In fact, God protects Cain from dying with the mark of protection. It seems that God loves Cain and exile is what Cain needs to do to restore himself to community with God.

Cain accepts the penance of this perpetual pilgrimage, and his wandering does not last forever, for he settles "east of Eden." This is an early, black-and-white snapshot of satisfaction. Cain accepts the punishment and he goes and does it. In the Bible we will see this same pattern again and again. It is as if it is embedded into the fabric of humanity.

Satisfaction is how we remember our sin. In satisfaction we are forced to remember it as we go on our penitential journey of restoration. By remembering it, we change the shame of it into something else—something we can live with. This takes time, which is why many penances involved walking to a specific place to pray. We can imagine Cain leaving the area of Eden and going east. With each step he remembers the rage he felt on that fateful day. He remembers how the rock felt in his hand. He remembers the horror that swept over him when he shook his brother's shoulder and said, "Are you okay?"

Cain remembers all this as he walks. And, as he walks, he feels the hard stones of the trail and the fiery sun burning his skin. He suffers the loss of his family and the loneliness pierces his heart. All this is mixed together, changing his shameful memory into a memory of guilt, suffering, and satisfaction. Cain accepted his punishment because there was a shred of hope in it.

After making a one-on-one confession to a priest or another Christian according to the rite of Reconciliation in the Book of Common Prayer, the penitent says,

Therefore, O Lord, from these and all other sins I cannot now remember, I turn to you in sorrow and repentance. Receive me again into the arms of your mercy and restore me to the blessed company of your faithful people; through him in whom you have redeemed the world, your Son our Savior Jesus Christ. Amen. —Book of Common Prayer, 450

THOUGHTS TO PONDER

1. Are you willing to do what it takes to experience reconciliation?

_____

_____

_____

2. Have you ever felt hopeless, but then felt a small shiver of hope?

_____

_____

_____

3. What are some other Bible stories that have a description of satisfaction in them?

_____

_____

_____

DAY 21 Steps taken: _____ Miles journeyed: _____

Exercise chosen: _____

Something I thought about: _____

_____

_____

_____

_____

Something I need to pray about: _____

_____

_____

_____

_____

What Is Penance?

BIBLICAL BIG IDEA #22

Peter replied, "Change your hearts and lives. Each of you must be baptized in the name of Jesus Christ for the forgiveness of your sins. Then you will receive the gift of the Holy Spirit." —Acts 2:38 (Common English Bible)

Me: Hey God?
God: Yes?
Me: Here's a quarter. Forgiven?
God: Yes and no. #itscomplicated

Penance is a punishment undergone in token of penitence for sin, connected to confession and repentance. Punishment is such an icky word, especially in today's society. Hence God's response, "#itscomplicated." Historically, people have seen penance as paying their way out of a sin, which in part led to the Reformation and the controversy of the merits of "faith" and "good works." Some people would think that if you wrote a check to the church, a magic wand is waved and *voila!* the sin goes away and salvation is assured. But it's not like that. Sure, you can pay a penance for your sins: enact forms of self-punishment, write checks, and do good deeds, but if your heart hasn't changed, then none of that matters. Like most things in the church, penance is an internal action of turning your heart back to God. Like many things, only God really sees if you are sincere about your penance and repentance. Other people may see the change in you through consistent, disciplined action towards making decisions that point you in the direction of God and away from your sin. "In penitence, we confess our sins and make restitution where possible, with the intention to amend our lives."[5]

---

5. Book of Common Prayer, 857.

But penance—is it important? Is it necessary? Progressive and modern theologians would probably say no. We can't buy our way back into God's grace or forgiveness any more than we can go on sinning and think it doesn't matter for our salvation. God's grace and forgiveness are freely given, but for whatever mysterious reason, we often continue to sin and keep repeating behaviors that separate us from God. And we wonder why it feels like we aren't receiving the grace and forgiveness of God anymore. Those actions, thoughts, feelings, traumas, and events that we are holding inside are like a brick wall for letting God's grace get through. Every action we take, every angry thought we percolate, every negative feeling we stoke, lays another brick in that wall. (Check out Pink Floyd's "Another Brick in the Wall"[6] and do some head-banging moves.) It's not God putting up a wall towards the way forward, it's us and what we do.

What does all this have to do with penance you may ask? Doing penance is like establishing a pattern of behaviors that you want to practice that will bring you closer to God. It's making amends. It's providing restitution for what was done wrong. In the Roman Catholic tradition, in response to your confessed sin, the priest tells you that you need to say ten "Our Fathers" every day for ten days. The penance isn't necessarily the "Our Father," the penance is establishing the pattern of prayer on a daily basis that will help you establish habits that bring you closer to God. The purpose of penance is not to buy our way back to God's presence (we never left it), but rather to do those things that help *us* realize we are there, we are forgiven, and we will always be worthy of God's love. Penance helps to put us back on the path God intends for us. Penance helps us to break down walls (cue some Pink Floyd again), giving us an action to take that will help us acknowledge we have strayed, but in our hearts we want to be back with God. Think of penance as a step in the reconciliation process to finding our way back to God by changing our hearts and lives.

When we are cross, angry, disgruntled, discombobulated, dis-this, and dis-that, it's often because we've lost our way. It's like picking up a cup of coffee to take a swig and realizing the cup is empty—you stare at it and wonder, "Where the heck is the coffee?" You've paused and

---

6. https://www.youtube.com/watch?v=pnbx00-L_EI (accessed September 20, 2018).

realized something is terribly wrong and you need to do something about it before you completely lose your mind. Filling your soul up with practices that bring you closer to God is like filling up an empty coffee cup. Once it's done, you can take a deep breath, smell the wonder, close your eyes in bliss, release the tension, and realize everything is going to be okay.

As you walk on today's journey, think about penance.

THOUGHTS TO PONDER

1. Is your coffee cup empty? (If you aren't a coffee drinker—God bless you—think of something else you enjoy with verve and imagine the cup or glass empty.)

_____

_____

_____

2. What can you do on a regular basis to "fill up"?

_____

_____

_____

3. Does the regular practice of this action bring you closer to God? If yes, how? If no, what "penance" can you do on a regular basis to bring you closer to God? What new habit, pattern, or repetition do you need to take on?

_____

_____

_____

DAY 22   Steps taken: _____   Miles journeyed: _____

Exercise chosen: _____

Something I thought about: _____

_____

_____

_____

_____

Something I need to pray about: _____

_____

_____

_____

_____

DAY 23 What Are Prayers of Sorrow?

BIBLICAL BIG IDEA #23

Likewise the Spirit also helpeth our infirmities: for we know not what we should pray for as we ought: but the Spirit itself maketh intercession for us with groanings which cannot be uttered. —Romans 8:26 (King James Version)

Meanwhile, the moment we get tired in the waiting, God's Spirit is right alongside helping us along. If we don't know how or what to pray, it doesn't matter. He does our praying in and for us, making prayer out of our wordless sighs, our aching groans. He knows us far better than we know ourselves, knows our pregnant condition, and keeps us present before God. That's why we can be so sure that every detail in our lives of love for God is worked into something good. —Romans 8:26–28 (The Message)

Me: Hey God?
God: Yes?
Me: Ugh. Uuuuuuuuuuuuuuuuugh. Gaaaaaaaaaaaaaah. Gasp.
God: Now you're talkin'.

There is a sound we hear that scares us when it comes out of another human's mouth. I remember hearing it in Iraq, when I was there as an Army chaplain. My convoy had just arrived at an Iraqi army base and, while we were climbing out of our vehicles, we saw an Iraqi soldier tearing his shirt, weeping, and groaning loudly. We were told he had just learned his brother had died. He wasn't speaking words, he was speaking in what St. Paul called, "groanings." I'll never forget that moment.

We like to say that cavemen (and cavewomen) communicated with grunts, as if it were a laughable way to communicate, but, if you've ever heard someone groan, you know exactly what they mean. You know exactly what they feel. And maybe God does too. Maybe God knows what our groans mean when we're curled up in a ball on the floor.

The prayer of sorrow, a response to the gravity of what we have done and left undone, is often written down. The all-time classic prayer of sorrow is Psalm 51, a poem written after King David's debacle with Bathsheba and Uriah.

The penitent king prayed, "For I know my transgressions, and my sin is ever before me. Against you, you alone, have I sinned, and done what is evil in your sight, so that you are justified in your sentence and blameless when you pass judgment" (Psalm 51:3–4). It's an honest prayer, a groan that has been translated into words.

It can happen when you have spoken your truth about what you have done and left undone. When you have felt the full weight of what others have done to you, sometimes all you can do is groan. And God hears us. God knows what we're saying.

THOUGHTS TO PONDER

1. If you're in a secured place, try groaning, either as a memory of a traumatic time or for a present distress.

_____

_____

_____

2. How does that feel?

_____

_____

_____

3. What do you think God feels when we groan? (There are no wrong answers.)

_____

_____

_____

DAY 23 Steps taken: _____ Miles journeyed: _____

Exercise chosen: _____

Something I thought about: _____

_____

_____

_____

_____

Something I need to pray about: _____

_____

_____

_____

_____

DAY 24 What Does It Mean to Reveal Truth?

BIBLICAL BIG IDEA #24

For the wrath of God is revealed from heaven against all ungodliness and wickedness of those who by their wickedness suppress the truth. —Romans 1:18

Me: Hey God?
God: Yes?
Me: I don't want to tell anyone what's in my heart.
God: Too bad. I want you to.

Truth-telling is putting into words your thoughts, feelings, and actions that got you where you are today. It is a bit of testimony, a bit of a spiritual autobiography, a bit of confession. Both David and I practice truth-telling whenever we go to talk about our books because we know that it is through the sharing of our stories that we touch other people who have been in similar shoes.

I remember sharing the story of my hearing loss at a women's retreat. It was incredibly painful, confusing, frustrating, and soul-defining to lose my hearing when I was fifteen. I was an awkward, sick, overweight teen with raging hormones on a cocktail of medications trying to fix what was wrong with me that had horrendous side effects, including mood swings. Did I mention that I was a hormone-raging teen? Already dealing with body self-loathing, self-consciousness, and pimples, I had to cope with massive prescription steroids, chemotherapy drugs, hair loss, stretch marks, depression, and a host of other issues (let's not forget the loss of my hearing). I was a mess in and out of the hospital. I hated everyone and everything, including myself and God. However, if there was ever a mystical experience in my life, it was being in church one Sunday bawling (hormone swing) and frustrated (hormone swing) and angry (hormone swing), and I couldn't hear the Eucharist. I sat down and refused to participate in the service. (Mind you, my father was the priest at the church and he was presiding over the Eucharist. Ask any preacher's kid—there are behaviors that are expected of you at church and sitting down, crying, and refusing to participate in worship isn't one of them.) In that moment God came to me. The angels sang, there was a cloud of the heavenly host, there was a person, the air shimmered, everything else dimmed and it was just me and God. Well, not really all that, but definitely a moment where there was just me and God. Nothing else. I definitely wasn't alone. And I did hear God speak to me. And it felt great. I remember I quit crying. All God said to me was that I didn't need to *hear* the Word of God—I needed to *live* the Word of God. Christianity isn't all about hearing, it is about living it and no amount of deafness could stop that.

This is one part of my reconciliation story. It's part of my truth-telling. It's important to share because there may be someone else out there who has felt that they were less than, less worthy, less able to participate in the Word of God because of a disability or illness and God wants them to know that's a bunch of hogwash. We aren't less this or less that in the eyes of God. You (and me and us) are *everything* in the eyes of God. There is a reason God seeks out and embraces the deaf, the blind, the poor, the meek, the hungry, the oppressed. It's easy to confuse physical wholeness with spiritual wholeness, but that's not what it's all about. God's calling *all of us* to *live* the Word of God, not just *hear* it.

Why do I tell you this? First, you might be one of those "less than" people who need to hear that, "Nope, you are more than enough. You are just right in God's eyes and there is plenty of your 'more than' for you to share with someone else." Second, both David and I want you to do some truth-telling for yourself. It's a large part of the reconciliation process to go and share your story. It's incredibly healing and a reminder of where you were, where you are, and where you want to go. The thing about truth-telling is it takes practice. The first time you tell your story, well, awkward doesn't begin to cover it. I still turn into a sweaty beast when I get up in front of a room and share my story. My heart races, my whole self sweats, and I feel a little sick. But as I get into my groove, I realize that God is working through me in those moments. In your moment of truth-telling, I guarantee God will be working through you, too, because somewhere, some place, and in some time, there is some-one who needs to hear your story.

Christ Walk Crushed was designed to be done by yourself or with a small group of faithful people trying to find their way back to God. It might be in these small groups that you find it easiest to tell your truth. The more you tell your truth, the easier it will be. And the thing about truth-telling is that it reveals God's faithfulness to all people. Love and grace flourish in the midst of truth-telling.

On today's journey think about what your truth-telling should be.

THOUGHTS TO PONDER

1. What's your truth?

_____

_____

_____

2. How does it make you feel to share that truth?

_____

_____

_____

3. Where is one place you think you could try sharing your truth?

_____

_____

_____

4. After you shared your truth, how did it go?

_____

_____

_____

DAY 24 Steps taken: _____ Miles journeyed: _____

Exercise chosen: _____

Something I thought about: _____

_____

_____

_____

_____

Something I need to pray about: _____

_____

_____

_____

_____

Are There Different Types of Penance?

BIBLICAL BIG IDEA #25

So the Philistines seized him and gouged out his eyes. They brought him down to Gaza and bound him with bronze shackles; and he ground at the mill in the prison. But the hair of his head began to grow again after it had been shaved.
—Judges 16:21–22

Me: Hey God?
God: Yeah?
Me: I got ants in my pants and nowhere to run.
God: Run to me.

The truth is, you're going to do it either way. After a loss, after a tragedy, after a personal failure, you're going feel the need to *do* something, even if it's hard to know why you're doing it.

Every weekend, thousands of people around the world run marathons, 5Ks, Tough Mudders, Spartan Races, and GORUCK events to suffer. These "suffer-fests" are not overtly religious, but they are often rituals of secular penance.

After Iraq and my personally traumatic divorce, I threw myself into running. I was so hyper-alert from untreated PTSD, I was constantly nauseous, and lost about thirty pounds. I would run about fifteen miles a day, morning and night, which gave me a sense I was moving toward something, even though I didn't know what it was. The day I ran the Boston Marathon was just another in a series of meaningless wanderings. I was on a penitential pilgrimage, but I didn't know it.

I've heard this same tale from so many people who have suffered—we need to take control of something, even if it's just the control of our feet, one step at a time. It is not a coincidence that modern people

97

engage in distance events and medieval people went on long pilgrimages after war and trauma. The human need to leave, pray, and come back are deep in our soul.

Samson, the man who is blinded and forced to grind wheat at the mill like an ox, is on a penitential pilgrimage. He is suffering for his own sins and the sins of others. With each step something changes inside him so that, in due time, he finds his true calling in one final, brave act of defiance to the invading Philistines.

I hope that your journey through this book is a kind of pilgrimage. I also trust you to construct your own pilgrimage route so you can make the conscious and unconscious journey toward reconciliation.

Another type of penance is saying prayers. When we repeat prayers out loud, we are engaging our bodies in prayer. If we stand up, walk, and pray, we are essentially in pilgrimage.

And, since it's hard to eat and run/walk or climb over obstacles, we naturally fast on pilgrimage. Fasting is simply giving something up, food, snacks, dinner, meat, or ice cream.

Pilgrimage unifies all penances, and so it is at the heart of our journey back to healing and wholeness. It is very physical. Penance does not ask you to change your mind about anything; it trusts your mind to adapt to your body, so that your mind will change gradually and of its own accord. Penance respects the will of the person and does not seek to impose a thought or feeling on someone who is resistant.

Even though pilgrimages end when we reach the destination, the life of pilgrimage never ends. This is why it works. We need short-term and long-term solutions to our pain and suffering. We need to go on a journey rather than just learn a magic spell. It's hard work out there on the road alone, but it is work worth doing.

THOUGHTS TO PONDER

1. What "pilgrimages" have you gone on unwittingly or unknowingly?

_____

_____

_____

2. What king of pilgrimage would fit with your particular issue or circumstance?

_____

_____

_____

3. Who do you know who has done such a thing?

_____

_____

_____

DAY 25 Steps taken: _____   Miles journeyed: _____

Exercise chosen: _____

Something I thought about: _____

_____

_____

_____

_____

Something I need to pray about: _____

_____

_____

_____

_____

DAY 26 Why Is Penance Important?

BIBLICAL BIG IDEA #26

Have mercy on me, O God, according to your steadfast love;
according to your abundant mercy blot out my transgressions.
—Psalm 51:1

Me: Hey God?
God: Yes?
Me: Have mercy on me, forgive my transgressions.
God: Done.

The experience of penance allows us to be open to the experience of God's grace and mercy. Mercy is the forgiveness and compassion we receive from those who have the power to withhold it. The whole story of Christ's crucifixion and resurrection is a story of God's mercy. By Jesus' obedience, even to suffering and death, Christ made the offering that we could not make; in him we are freed from the power of sin and reconciled to God.[7] God always wants us to find our way back to God. The gift of Christ's resurrection is the promise that God will make all whole for all of us. Reconciliation ensures that each of us opens our hearts to that gift. Penance is simply a part of that reconciliation process.

For whatever crazy human reason we might have, it seems unfathomable to us that God could continue to repeatedly forgive us for our sins. We keep messing up and God keeps saying, "I'm here! Come back!" Over and over and over again as this cycle happens God is ever faithful and ever present. Practicing penance challenges us to demonstrate that same level of compassion and forgiveness with others.

---

7. From "The Outline of the Faith" in the Book of Common Prayer, 850.

With penance, if what is separating ourselves from God is an issue with someone else, God is going to call us to dig deep for compassion for and reconciliation with that other person. This can feel like punishment, especially when we are really angry with another person. It's a lot easier to hold on to animosity for another person than to demonstrate clemency, tolerance, and grace. But this is exactly what God expects us to do. God's steadfast love is for everyone, and sometimes that mercy and compassion come through you.

When you hold on to hatred, self-righteousness, and bitterness, a physical burden is placed on your body. Your body becomes stressed from mental and spiritual anguish: your heart beats at a faster resting heart rate; it may feel difficult to catch your breath; your blood pressure may become chronically elevated, which puts stress on your heart. You begin to produce cortisone hormones because your biological systems believe they are in a constant state of flight and are preparing for the body to be attacked again. Your body thinks you are under assault and this has a very real physical manifestation. It is difficult for your body to recover from this emotional trauma.

Maybe your penance is to let go of all this. Maybe it is to practice mindful behaviors and feelings of empathy and charity, even to those who might not deserve it. As my mom says to me, "Deserve's got nothing to do with it." We are called to practice the same mercy, forgiveness, and compassion that God shows to each of us. This practice is important because it's *healthy* for mind, body, and spirit; research demonstrates that those who practice the cycle of reconciliation/forgiveness have positive health benefits and are more at peace.[8] These *feelings* result in very physical responses such as lowered heart rate and blood pressure, stabilization of hormone fluctuations, and others. These physical and emotion responses are the result of your spirit healing and feeling at balance with God. This is our spiritual communion with our maker. It is a process of both action and acceptance. It is not passive. If you want to be a part of the reconciliation cycle both with God and with others, you'll need to get involved and take action. Hence, penance.

---

8. A. H. S. Harris and C. E. Thoresen (2005). "Forgiveness, Unforgiveness, Health, and Disease" in E. L. Worthington, Jr. (editor), *Handbook of Forgiveness* (New York: Brunner-Routledge, 2005), 321–334.

On today's journey, I want you to think about the importance of receiving God's mercy.

THOUGHTS TO PONDER

1. Where can you demonstrate mercy, compassion, and forgiveness in your life?

_____

_____

_____

2. Where are you demonstrating areas of anger, bitterness, and self-righteousness?

_____

_____

_____

3. Where do you need to find balance?

_____

_____

_____

DAY 26 Steps taken: _____ Miles journeyed: _____

Exercise chosen: _____

Something I thought about: _____

_____

_____

_____

_____

Something I need to pray about: _____

_____

_____

_____

_____

DAY 27 Why Do Penance When the Injury Was Done to Us?

BIBLICAL BIG IDEA #27

The priest shall take some of the blood of the sin offering and put it on the doorposts of the temple, the four corners of the ledge of the altar, and the posts of the gate of the inner court. You shall do the same on the seventh day of the month for anyone who has sinned through error or ignorance; so you shall make atonement for the temple. —Ezekiel 45:19–20

Me: Hey God?

God: Yes?

Me: If Jesus is the perfect son of God, why did he get baptized? And also, can you please put out that cigar? It's making me cough.

God: Why are you coughing? I'm the one smoking it.

I admit it, I've been talking out of two sides of my mouth to you. On the one hand I've been dropping some knowledge on how to find reconciliation through contrition, repentance, penance, et cetera, after you have "erred and strayed from thy ways like lost sheep."[9] On the other hand, I've been trying to walk alongside you as you recover from the things other people did to you. I have not been as clear as I could have, so I'll state it plainly: DON'T REPENT OF THINGS OTHER PEOPLE DID TO YOU! Can I shout it again? Okay. You've got it.

When other people sin against us, or something "happens" to us (like a disease or a natural disaster), this is not the main material we bring

---

9. This is from the prayer of confession found in Morning Prayer, Rite I, Book of Common Prayer, 41.

to God in the practices and rituals of reconciliation. However, there's a plot twist. For many of us, it was these exterior injuries, oppressions, abuses, and diseases that came from the outside and planted the bitter seeds that led to our moral injuries and sins in later months and years. Many of us breathed the second-hand smoke of someone else's smoking habit.

I hope my story illustrates this point. My experiences of war in Iraq and the divorce when I came home aren't sins I need to repent of. But, these massively life-changing experiences wounded my mind and spirit and those wounds were easily infected. So, the stuff I bring to confession, the things I do penance for, are often my attempts to fix the bad stuff that happened to me. These actions were often unintentional, like the inadvertent sins mentioned in the biblical big idea above. But their involuntary nature did not exclude them from the need for atonement and reconciliation. In the deep fabric of the universe there is a need for healing and reconciliation for every tiny thing that has gone wrong, no matter the reason it went wrong.

I grew up in the age of participation trophies, which are easily mocked these days. But there is a truth about the participation trophy—that is, when we participate in a sport, the sport participates in us. When I participated in war, war participated in me. To parse out the complications of how much is "my fault" or the fault of others is often vital for healing and should be done over time with a competent therapist and counselor.

Penance is a broad-brush approach to healing. It's a full immersion into a healing journey. When treating one particular sin or moral injury through penance, I often find healing in other areas of my life. If this is confusing, forgive me. I just want you to know that you should never do penance for something that was done to you. However, when you do penance for the things "done and left undone," I suspect those other wounds in your life will find some healing too.

In the Book of Common Prayer there is a cryptic line in Form Two of the rite called Reconciliation of a Penitent[10] that I don't fully understand. After the penitent has confessed the particulars of the sin and right before the priest pronounces absolution, the priest asks, "Do you,

---

10. "The Reconciliation of a Penitent" (Form One and Form Two) can be found in the Book of Common Prayer beginning on page 446.

then, forgive those who have sinned against you?" The answer, if given, is "I forgive them." This is a clear reminder that so many of our sins are reactions to the evils of others or the evils of the world. It points to the deeper truth that to live on this planet in human flesh is to participate in sin's second-hand smoke.

Some military vehicles have "reactive armor." When an enemy projectile hits the reactive armor, the armor explodes so the force of its blast will counter the force of the enemy's projectile. The blast from the reactive armor has the potential to wound people around it. We are all covered in layers of reactive armor. As we rightfully and legitimately protect ourselves, we often blast some of the bystanders around us. This is why we bring *all* these things to God.

THOUGHTS TO PONDER

1. Have you spoken with a therapist about what was done to you?

_____

_____

_____

2. Are there any complicated people in movies you relate to?

_____

_____

_____

DAY 27 Steps taken: _____ Miles journeyed: _____

Exercise chosen: _____

Something I thought about: _____

_____

_____

_____

_____

Something I need to pray about: _____

_____

_____

_____

_____

DAY 28 How Do I Make Things Right?

BIBLICAL BIG IDEA #28

For just as by the one man's disobedience the many were made sinners, so by the one man's obedience the many will be made righteous. —Romans 5:19

Me: Hey God?
God: Yes?
Me: I'm righteous, man!
God: No, I'm righteous, you need to be obedient.

Obedience to God creates conflict in our lives. Humans have a tendency towards self-righteousness that has nothing to do with God. God wants us to be obedient: love yourself, love your neighbor. Are you failing at this today? It's easy to do; on a weekly basis I can hate myself and others fairly easily. It's a lot harder to practice the pause button in order to first think about loving someone else and myself no matter what has happened. God calls me to be far more than what I can do on my own.

On your journey towards reconciliation, you may need to make things right. I like to think of this as loving my neighbor. Along the way you may have intentionally, or unintentionally, done things that hurt someone. It's incredibly healing to ask forgiveness for what you have done or not done to another person. Just as we ask forgiveness of God, it's often important to ask forgiveness of others. It's a step in the journey towards wholeness to acknowledge that you could have done something differently, opening up the possibility for doing those things another way in the future. We are always on a journey of becoming better Christians, because there is no such thing as a perfect Christian.

Say you've made this step towards making things right. You are on your quest for healing, wholeness, and reconciliation with God. You are striving for the balance, the new you, the joy, and the peace that comes with making a change in your life. You *want* things to be different. You've acknowledged that things need to change, you are ready to let go of your hurts and injuries and move on, and you are taking great strides in making an effort towards those changes. You've come to this place where you've taken a deep breath, said a little prayer. and told the person you've offended the magic words, "I'm sorry." (Internally wave a magic wand.)

Nothing happens. Maybe the person you've asked forgiveness of tells you off, walks away, or, in some ways worse, doesn't respond at all (which has happened to me). You've gone to this great effort and you are left holding a bag of forgiveness that was thrown back in your face. What now?

Some people won't forgive you for whatever you've done. That's when you have to realize that God and the world are two different things and we need to accept God's forgiveness even if someone else won't. You can't make someone else forgive you. That's their journey. You've done what you could to make things right; your journey towards reconciliation is not dependent on the actions of others. It's between you and God at the end of the day. Being obedient to God's will for us is to try to make things right, which is part of the journey. I really don't think you'll find the peace and joy you seek without acknowledging those areas on your journey where you need to ask forgiveness. Do it, and then if someone else doesn't accept it, it's on them, not you.

If anyone refuses to welcome you or listen to your words, shake the dust off your feet as you leave that house or town. —Matthew 10:14

On today's journey, think about obedience. To God.

THOUGHTS TO PONDER

1. What are some things you feel like you need to ask forgiveness for?

_____

_____

_____

2. Who do you need to engage with to ask forgiveness?

_____

_____

_____

3. Why is it an important part of your journey?

_____

_____

_____

4. How do you think it's going to go?

_____

_____

_____

5. (After you ask forgiveness:) What happened?

_____

_____

_____

DAY 28 Steps taken: _____ Miles journeyed: _____

Exercise chosen: _____

Something I thought about: _____

_____

_____

_____

_____

Something I need to pray about: _____

_____

_____

_____

_____

How Do We Let Go of Sin?

BIBLICAL BIG IDEA #29

Therefore, since we are surrounded by so great a cloud of witnesses, let us also lay aside every weight and the sin that clings so closely, and let us run with perseverance the race that is set before us, looking to Jesus the pioneer and perfecter of our faith, who for the sake of the joy that was set before him endured the cross, disregarding its shame, and has taken his seat at the right hand of the throne of God.
—Hebrews 12:1–2

Me: Hey God?

God: Yes?

Me: That song from the movie *Frozen* is really annoying.

God: Actually, I kinda like it.

It seems like a distant memory now, but during my deployment to Iraq I wore armor, lots of it. It was heavy and the Iraqi sun made it nearly unbearable. After that experience, I can testify there is no better feeling in the world than taking off that armor.

I've also carried packs, weights at the gym, and tired toddlers after a long day at the park, and so have you. There is truly no better metaphor in the world than to "let something go."

But where we let something go is just as important as when we let something go. The guilt, shame, and burdens we carry have a way of jumping back into our packs and arms. Like Frodo, we must cast them into the fires of Mount Doom, from whence they came.

Jesus did this in his life, death, and resurrection. Jesus travels light, with no place to call his own. He does not get married and have children, he owns nothing but a garment, and he refuses to amass wealth, weapons, or status. He asks others to travel light too, to leave their fishing nets and money tables, and follow him. On the cross he is naked; his only possessions are a crown of thorns, four nails, and the sins of the whole world. And then he gives up his spirit. He's put in a tomb, and the next thing we see is him leaving his burial shroud behind! He's laying everything down—he's letting it all go.

Jesus is telling us that God is spirit and if we are to worship this spirit-god, we must do so in spirit and in truth. Traumatic experiences have a way of stripping away our material comforts. World-changing experiences have a way of showing us how hollow possessions are, and how wealth will not solve all our problems.

And so, to let something go is not a good thing we can do, it is the only thing we can do. There is an old proverb that says, "People don't tell you of their troubles unless they are fond of them." Take that however you want it, but I can confess I am invested in my troubles. I sometimes wonder who I would be if you took them away.

Jesus calls us to come to him if we are weary and heavy laden. He will give us rest. We need to let things go if we are to walk, run, live, or love. Letting things go is a prerequisite to really living.

THOUGHTS TO PONDER

1. What is one thing you've left behind that gave you freedom?

_____

_____

_____

2. Are there other things you need to leave behind?

_____

_____

_____

DAY 29   Steps taken: _____   Miles journeyed: _____

Exercise chosen: _____

Something I thought about: _____

_____

_____

_____

_____

Something I need to pray about: _____

_____

_____

_____

_____

What Actions
Do We Take during
Satisfaction?

BIBLICAL BIG IDEA #30
*I consider that the sufferings of this present time are not
worth comparing with the glory about to be revealed to us.*
—Romans 8:18

Me: Hey God?

God: Yes?

Me: Can't. Let. This. Go.

God: Funny. I did. If I didn't let go of everything humans did
wrong, we'd never get anywhere. Remember when I said,
"as far from the east is from the west"? That's what you need
to think when you repent. Time to move on.[11]

The idea behind satisfaction is you've paid your price for your sin. Whatever it is, whatever is separating yourself from God and whatever you've done to bring yourself back into communion with God, and you are striving each day away from sinful practices and towards those things that bring you closer to God. . . then, you move on. You don't stay penitent forever. God always says, "Go." God always has something else in store for you. God is always trying to work you towards a process of wholeness.

Think of it like this: Both David and I ran races during our reconciliation (wrestling with God) periods. Contrition is the step where we acknowledge we need to do something. Things cannot go on as they have been before. The path, the journey, the road we are on needs to

11. See Psalm 103.

change and we need a new map to get there. Think of your training plan as your map of behavior change that helps you towards the goal. Its development puts you on the path towards repentance and towards the life (end goal) you want. Metaphorically, God is the "big finish line" you are seeking toward wholeness. Each additional mile is a bit of penance. Not only do the extra miles stretch you physically, but there is pain associated with the steps needed to be taken to get you to where you want to be.

I remember vividly thinking that I was squashing my cancer cells, anxiety, and anger under my running shoe. I'd listen for the pounding of my foot into the ground. I remember my teeth grinding, and with each breath I imagined expelling all the bad that was in my body at the time. If you don't experience penance with running, you aren't running far enough. Ha! The idea is to push yourself just enough to make yourself stronger. Each step is one step closer to God. It's one more repetitious step towards disciplined behavior. Satisfaction is finishing the race, not giving up no matter how hard, slow, or painful things get. While there are no medals in the process of reconciliation, satisfaction can be likened to paying the entrance fee of a marathon so that you get your medal when you cross the finish line. You want to see God at that finish line and that means pulling up the big girl (or boy) britches and getting it done.

Absolution is the joy we feel when we have accomplished our goal. As much as I have a love/hate relationship with running, there is nothing quite like finishing a race. I've run both good and bad races. Even the bad races give me a sense of accomplishment. We feel right with God and are balanced yet again in our mind, body, and spiritual practices. Hopefully along those miles we've let go of the pain of our injury, abuse, or illness. I don't believe that you ever really get rid of these events in your life that caused you moral injury, but I think that it changes. It crops up from time to time, but when you have a training plan, you know how to deal with it when it rears its ugly head. The sacrament of reconciliation is giving you a process or framework in which to deal with spiritual injury in a healthy way. Sometimes the race doesn't get completed. That's when you need to relook at your training plan and see what's missing. Remember, this is a process and evolves over time as you learn things about yourself, your body, your mind, and what you really need. I thought for years I needed to run but have since learned differently. There are a lot of ways towards a healthy life; reconciliation helps you figure it all out.

Do you have to run? Not at all. You can take any sort of journey during the practice of reconciliation but with *Christ Walk Crushed*, we're putting miles towards those steps so that you can see the output of your effort. We do highly recommend some sort of physical exercise because it's a healthy habit and the benefits of activity when you've been dealt a sorry hand of cards are well documented. When you track the miles you can see how far you've come in the process.

To this day, David continues to run as part of his practice. I do a lot of different things with exercise and fitness in general and have found that I am able to connect more deeply to my spiritual self through yoga and walking. My practice changed over time with amazing benefits to my life. Your practice my change over time too and that's okay. Even if your training plan shifts a bit, you still have the keys to getting yourself back on track.

I wish I could say that once you experience one traumatic event you've paid your dues for a lifetime, but alas, that's not the way the world works. Garbage has a way of stalking people. Sin has a way of creeping up on you. Hopefully, with *Christ Walk Crushed* you are gaining tools to make you stronger when the inevitable happens. Maybe you'll even see the joy in these moments as well. Whatever happens, all it takes is one step to get you back to God.

THOUGHTS TO PONDER

1. Have you run your race with perseverance?

_____

_____

_____

2. Where are you on your journey?

_____

_____

_____

3. Do you need to adjust your training plan?

_____

_____

_____

4. Are you ready to let go of your sin and move on?

_____

_____

_____

DAY 30   Steps taken: _____   Miles journeyed: _____

Exercise chosen: _____

Something I thought about: _____

_____

_____

_____

_____

Something I need to pray about: _____

_____

_____

_____

_____

What Is Absolution?

BIBLICAL BIG IDEA #31

Then the disciples rejoiced when they saw the Lord. Jesus said to them again, "Peace be with you. As the Father has sent me, so I send you." When he had said this, he breathed on them and said to them, "Receive the Holy Spirit. If you forgive the sins of any, they are forgiven them; if you retain the sins of any, they are retained." —John 20:20b–23

Me: Hey God?
God: Yes?
Me: . . .
God: . . .

I love hats. I have since my childhood and, when I reflect on my life choices, most of them have involved hats. As I write this, I must remind you I grew up in the '80s, when hats were definitely not in fashion. The towering bangs on women's foreheads and the permed mullets on men precluded hats. Occasionally, baseball hats were seen, but not much else.

And so, when I was eight, I made a top hat out of paper and wore it all the time. I must also admit the cool hats of the Marine Corps were a big draw for me, and I joined the Army just as the black beret was authorized for all personnel.

Now that I work at a church, I have a small but beloved churchy hat collection. Whenever we have an outdoor procession, you'll likely see me wearing one. For some reason I can't quite fathom, these hats evoke significant responses in people. Some of these responses are critical, as if I am trying to impose my theology on them through my hat. I always tell my critics I'm wearing the hat because I really like hats. Sometimes, my response to is: "You should have seen the hats I wore in the military. Those were weird hats!"

My favorite hat is probably the biretta, a hat that looks like a little Russian church dome. It's black and has a little happy pom-pom that lives on its top. (Google it now and my picture will likely come up.)

The biretta is an old hat mainly worn by Roman Catholic and Anglo-Catholic priests. In reading about this unusual cap, I stumbled on a very strange use of it in England and Europe. In many places, judges would don their biretta one time during the trial, to pronounce the sentence of death. This is a chilling scene to imagine, as it becomes rarer and rarer in our world. This cap signified the authority to send someone to the executioner.

When a priest stands up after the congregation says a general confession, that priest is kind of like that judge, but in reverse. The judge is declaring the death sentence on behalf of the state (and sometimes on behalf of God), whereas the priest or minister is standing up and pronouncing forgiveness and absolution on behalf of God.

While Christians have understood this differently over the years, the Bible is clear that Jesus forgave sins, and expected his disciples to do the same. He empowered them for this by breathing on them. Unlike medieval knighting ceremonies with a sword on each shoulder, Jesus breathed on his apostles, just as God breathed into Adam the breath of life at the beginning of our human story.

During the late Middle Ages, many Christians felt the priests had too much power. One of the ways to reduce that power was to remove their power to absolve sins. But it was the abuse of clergy power that made this practice problematic, not the practice itself. In my Episcopal tradition, priests are given special lines after a sin is confessed, but then we have a declaration of forgiveness that all Christians can say to a person who is penitent. We have this power! You have this power! It amazes me that many people in my church have never seen these pages in our prayer book:

Our Lord Jesus Christ, who offered himself to be sacrificed for us to the Father, forgives your sins by the grace of the Holy Spirit. Amen.[12]

I think there are many ways to find absolution, the declaration of the removal and forgiveness of sins. In some ways, I hope this book will

---

12. Book of Common Prayer, 448.

help you to realize the absolution that comes from God. I can imagine people finding absolution by going back to the person they wronged and hearing a kind word. I can imagine a long hike where a beautiful sunset says, you are loved, you are forgiven. But, many times, the person we wronged doesn't speak to us anymore, or the sunset isn't that specific. I still need someone to tell me this. I need someone to lay their hand on my head and tell me my sins are forgiven. I sometimes even need to see that judge-like figure with the silly hat on wave her hands and say, "Almighty God have mercy on you, forgive you all your sins through our Lord Jesus Christ, strengthen you in all goodness, and by the power of the Holy Spirit keep you in eternal life. *Amen.*"[13]

Remember, the power of absolution comes from God, just like every spiritual grace comes from God. But God has made us vessels to carry that grace and we all need to declare God's forgiveness to a world that needs to hear it.

As you walk or run today, remember that God wants to forgive you and absolve you. God wants to do this so much God sent Jesus to commission a brigade of "absolvers" to go into the world, with hats or without hats, to declare this absolution to you.

THOUGHTS TO PONDER

1. Have you ever experienced this, someone telling you are forgiven?

_____

_____

_____

2. When you imagine doing this, what feelings does it evoke in you?

_____

_____

_____

13. Book of Common Prayer, 360.

DAY 31   Steps taken: _____   Miles journeyed: _____

Exercise chosen: _____

Something I thought about: _____

_____

_____

_____

_____

Something I need to pray about: _____

_____

_____

_____

_____

How Long Do Absolution and Reconciliation Take?

BIBLICAL BIG IDEA #32

And the LORD *said to Moses, "How long will this people despise me? And how long will they refuse to believe in me, in spite of all the signs that I have done among them?*
—Numbers 14:11

Me: Hey God?
God: Yes?
Me: How long is this going to take?
God: As long as necessary.

How's your journey going? Think about how far you've come and how far you need to go. How long is that going to take? There is no magic number. Everyone's journey takes the amount of time they need to traverse their road. Grief isn't a set period of days and you get over it. As strong as I was going in to my cancer diagnosis, if I'm honest, it took me close to three years to feel more like myself again. Even now, I'm a different version of myself than I was before. There will be a "before" version of you and the "after" version of you. I don't think one who experiences a moral injury can stay the same or go back. The nature of spiritual, moral, and soul injury is transformative. You are never quite the same and that isn't necessarily a bad thing.

How long will this take? As long as necessary. Don't rush; you need to grieve about what happened to you. You need to acknowledge what you went through in order to move on. You need to say you hurt. I remember during my process that a friend told me I needed to get on with things; I was told I needed to let the guilt go. On the one hand, I really appreciated the kick in the rear. Things like this can often help you to recognize that things need to change, but on the other hand I was ticked off. I felt like I was being told it wasn't okay to be angry, guilty, depressed, and scared. I was told by a therapist (if you can believe it) that I wasn't trusting in God enough and was a weak Christian. There was this perception that if I just snapped my fingers I would get over what I was feeling and move on.

I disagree. I needed to feel what I felt and the time to work through and process what was happening, which included being angry. I think it would have been far unhealthier to bottle it all up and slap a smiley face on it all. None of this happens overnight. *Christ Walk Crushed* might be forty days long, but it doesn't mean that it ends there. It might take you longer while another person might take five days. Someone else might need to take this journey three or four or five times to get where they need to be. All this is good. There is nothing wrong with how long it takes to make change as long as you are working on it. It's when we aren't trying and instead wallowing in destructive behaviors that intervention is needed.

Generally speaking, it takes around six weeks to establish a *pattern* of healthy behavior. This is getting into the groove of the discipline. It can take up to six months for this habit to be normal for you. This is called maintenance. It can take even longer to where it feels normal. And then there can be relapse. Did you know that on average it takes a smoker four to five tries to quit smoking before the habit sticks? Processes of behavior change and recovery are similar. Relapse may happen. Sin might happen again (and probably will). We might get sloppy in our spiritual practices, so we'll need to apply the training program again. Falling back into bad habits happens, but that doesn't mean that it has to happen forever. *You have the tools* to get yourself back on track no matter how many times you wander.

THINGS TO PONDER:

1. Where are you on your journey?

_____

_____

_____

2. Do you feel like you are making progress?

_____

_____

_____

3. Have you relapsed?   Yes   No

4. If yes, are you ready to get back on track?

_____

_____

_____

DAY 32   Steps taken: _____   Miles journeyed: _____

Exercise chosen: _____

Something I thought about: _____

_____

_____

_____

_____

Something I need to pray about: _____

_____

_____

_____

_____

DAY 33 What Does Absolution Feel Like?

BIBLICAL BIG IDEA #33

Jesus said, "Which is easier, to say to the paralytic, 'Your sins are forgiven,' or to say, 'Stand up and take your mat and walk'? But so that you may know that the Son of Man has authority on earth to forgive sins"—he said to the paralytic— "I say to you, stand up, take your mat and go to your home." And he stood up, and immediately took the mat and went out before all of them; so that they were all amazed and glorified God, saying, "We have never seen anything like this!"
—Mark 2:9–12

Me: Hey God?
God: Yes?
Me: What does absolution feel like?
God: There's only one way to find out.

I hesitate to share this story, for fear you will think I am a bad priest. It's a story about a confession I heard, so I assure you that all of the details of the story are changed so much that the story may not make sense. The seal of the confessional is inviolate, not only to inquiring minds, but also to the person who is confessing. I will never bring up to you what you have brought up to God. I'll never see you walking down the street and whisper, "Hey, how is that 'problem' working out for you?" I won't go there because God doesn't go there.

So, this is the story. I met a couple in a random encounter while I was out walking while wearing my cassock (a priestly garment). We chit-chatted and I took their picture near a landmark. About a year later one of the couple contacted me and asked if they could talk with me. The only day they could meet was my day off, so I suggested a coffee shop near where I used to live.

We met at the busy coffee shop, amidst the open iMacs and young people who wore wool beanies even though it was quite warm out. I wore a t-shirt and shorts since it was my day off and I had biked over. Immediately, they were shocked I wasn't wearing my cassock, and said they wished I had. Okay, I thought, and we kept talking. Then they shared the reason they wanted to talk to me. You see, they had killed someone many years before and finished a lengthy prison sentence for the crime. The person wanted to do the Sacrament of Reconciliation right then and there, then had to get back to work.

I was flabbergasted. I had not expected this and didn't have a prayer book with me (a petty concern, I know, but I wanted to get the words right). So I pulled out my iPad and went to my electronic prayer book and we read out our parts right there among the hipsters. At the end there's a rubric, an instruction, that says "The Priest then lays a hand upon the penitent's head. . . ." So I did, right then and there. I said the absolution quickly, because I knew my hand on this person's head was going to give some folks whiplash when they turned to look at us.

And then it was over. We went our separate ways and we've never spoken again. In the category of "serious sins," that one was way up there, and in the category of "worst places to hear a confession" it was way up there, but maybe that's what we both needed that day. I know I needed to not take myself too seriously as a priest. After all, it is God's grace that worked through me, not any grace of my own. It wasn't my cassock, my church building, or my leather-bound prayer book that gave this person absolution—it was God.

The paralytic man whom Jesus forgives as well as physically heals demonstrates there is a physical dimension to all this. It was my hand on the penitent's head that became the conduit of grace, and truly nothing else.

So, what does absolution feel like? Absolution feels like a hand on your head. That's all I know.

THOUGHTS TO PONDER

1. What would be your ideal setting for saying or hearing a confession?

_____

_____

_____

2. What are the gestures of forgiveness your family practiced when you were a child?

_____

_____

_____

DAY 33 Steps taken: _____ Miles journeyed: _____

Exercise chosen: _____

Something I thought about: _____

_____

_____

_____

_____

Something I need to pray about: _____

_____

_____

_____

_____

Why Are the Steps on Our Journey Important to Absolution?

BIBLICAL BIG IDEA #34

Therefore, since we are surrounded by so great a cloud of witnesses, let us also lay aside every weight and the sin that clings so closely, and let us run with perseverance the race that is set before us, looking to Jesus the pioneer and perfecter of our faith, who for the sake of the joy that was set before him endured the cross, disregarding its shame, and has taken his seat at the right hand of the throne of God.
—Hebrews 12:1–2

Me: Hey God?
God: Yes?
Me: I'm tired.
God: Don't give up now. You've come so far.

Think about the steps you've taken and the steps you still plan to take. Steps and goals are markers on the way toward health and healing or any pilgrimage you may be on. They can represent penance, the process, the rebuilding of the broken temple (the body), the journey towards a new path with God. These steps are important. Documenting these steps on your journey is essential as well because when we are in the thick of dealing with our spiritual hurts, it's hard to see that we are making any progress at all. Writing down the small stuff adds up to big stuff long term. You might not see the progress now, but the documentation of your journey will make a big deal as you keep going.

THOUGHTS TO PONDER

1. Note one small thing you feel that you've accomplished:

_____

_____

_____

2. Note another small thing you feel that you've accomplished:

_____

_____

_____

3. Note a third thing you feel that you've accomplished:

_____

_____

_____

4. Does that add up to something bigger?

_____

_____

_____

DAY 34 Steps taken: _____ Miles journeyed: _____

Exercise chosen: _____

Something I thought about: _____

_____

_____

_____

_____

Something I need to pray about: _____

_____

_____

_____

_____

What Are the Benefits of Absolution from a Clergyperson?

BIBLICAL BIG IDEA #35

Since, then, we have a great high priest who has passed through the heavens, Jesus, the Son of God, let us hold fast to our confession. For we do not have a high priest who is unable to sympathize with our weaknesses, but we have one who in every respect has been tested as we are, yet without sin. Let us therefore approach the throne of grace with boldness, so that we may receive mercy and find grace to help in time of need. —Hebrews 4:14–16

Me: Hey God?

God: Yes?

Me: What was your plan for this whole mess down here?

God: Well, here's the master plan: First, I send Jesus to be born in a hostile environment, he picks twelve people, and only one of them betrays him. . . .

We must admit, in hindsight, God's plan of redemption never had much hope. God's insistence on working through the flawed lives of patriarchs, prophets, disciples, and apostles would be comical if it wasn't so tragic. Only a few characters in the Bible are free from glaring character deficiencies and poor judgment, and yet, this is the method, over and over again, for how God plans to save the world.

A member of the clergy is just as frail as these characters. We are just like you, full of anxieties and hopes. I am petty and vain, with an ego that is easily bruised. I try to rise above the negativity, but I often succumb to its downward gravity.

Clergypersons are sinners, saved by grace, but still sinners. We have cheated, lied, betrayed, stolen, and done far worse than this short list.

Not a day goes by without another priest, pastor, or minister making the news for doing something awful. And yet, God does not use these people in spite of their failings, God uses them in the midst of their shortcomings. This is a great mystery: how caring and loving we can be at times and how base and vile we can be at other times.

Absolution from a clergyperson isn't necessary to find reconciliation and forgiveness, but it personalizes this moment in time in a way that is not easily replicated. God is a personal God, sending a very personal son, Jesus, and breathing into us the Holy Spirit that knows our groans and sighs. We must be personal with each other, both in times of joy and times of penitence.

In the drama of salvation, as described above in the Letter to the Hebrews, we see Jesus acting in his priestly ministry. He looks strange to us in this role. He is no longer the poor, wandering rabbi, but an ancient priest passing through the heavens to serve in the heavenly temple. And he is just like us. He can sympathize with our weaknesses because he feels them, too.

This is true of his representatives here on earth also. Clergypersons can sympathize with your weaknesses, because we are weak too. And clergy are nobody special, let me tell you. The word "clergy" is related to the word "dice," since priests were selected by casting lots back in the day.

God comes to us in the person of Jesus Christ as well as in the followers of Jesus Christ. Perhaps God is calling you to becoming a part of the clergy order? Perhaps God is calling you to speak with a clergyperson about what you are experiencing? If you do, find a weak one to talk to, for they will be the most like Jesus.

THOUGHTS TO PONDER

1. What stereotypes of clergypersons do you carry with you from childhood?

---

2. Have you ever wondered if God is calling you to a more specialized form of ministry?

_____

_____

_____

DAY 35 Steps taken: _____ Miles journeyed: _____

Exercise chosen: _____

Something I thought about: _____

_____

_____

_____

_____

Something I need to pray about: _____

_____

_____

_____

_____

Will We Need Absolution Again?

BIBLICAL BIG IDEA #36

Absolve, O LORD, your people Israel, whom you redeemed; do not let the guilt of innocent blood remain in the midst of your people Israel. Then they will be absolved of bloodguilt.— Deuteronomy 21:8

Me: Hey God?
God: Yes?
Me: I screwed up again.
God: I know. And you'll probably do it again, and again, and again.

At some point you'll probably find yourself in a state again where you need forgiveness. It's the nature of individuals to mess up. That's why we pray (as part of the General Confession in the Episcopal Church) for forgiveness of those things done and left undone, or for those things we did without knowing we were causing offense. We acknowledge the fact that we are sinful creatures that are only saved through God's loving grace, and it is for this grace that we strive to repent and reconcile ourselves. The process of reconciliation is a cycle because we come and go through the stages of recognizing our behavior is not desired through different points in our life depending on what has happened to us. We cannot know the future and therefore we will most likely need a process in which to find redemption at every stage of our development.

It is comforting to know that there is always a path back to God no matter how many times I stray. I don't think of this as a pass to do whatever I want and then haphazardly repent each time. Rather, I look at it as a goal: trying hard each day to live your life as a child of God. It's inevitable that something will happen either intentionally or unintentionally that messes with the "love your God, love your neighbor" commandment. I know God is constantly working with me to live in a state of godly existence. It is in this state that we find joy and peace. I know that *when* I am following God's rules rather than my own I am obedient to something much better, stronger, wiser, and more faithful. Generally, I feel most people benefit from some type of obedience and discipline to something better than themselves.

In Psalm 103, King David (not our David, the other biblical David) gives thanks for God's everlasting goodness, mercy and forgiveness:

Bless the Lord, O my soul,
and all that is within me,
bless his holy name.
Bless the Lord, O my soul,
and do not forget all his benefits—
who forgives all your iniquity,
who heals all your diseases,
who redeems your life from the Pit,
who crowns you with steadfast love and mercy,
who satisfies you with good as long as you live
so that your youth is renewed like the eagle's.
The Lord works vindication
and justice for all who are oppressed.
He made known his ways to Moses,
his acts to the people of Israel.
The Lord is merciful and gracious,
slow to anger and abounding in steadfast love.
He will not always accuse,
nor will he keep his anger for ever.
He does not deal with us according to our sins,
nor repay us according to our iniquities.
For as the heavens are high above the earth,
so great is his steadfast love toward those who fear him;
as far as the east is from the west,
so far he removes our transgressions from us.
As a father has compassion for his children,
so the Lord has compassion for those who fear him.
For he knows how we were made;
he remembers that we are dust.

As for mortals, their days are like grass;
*   they flourish like a flower of the field;*
for the wind passes over it, and it is gone,
*   and its place knows it no more.*
But the steadfast love of the Lord is from everlasting to everlasting
*   on those who fear him,*
*   and his righteousness to children's children,*
to those who keep his covenant
*   and remember to do his commandments.*
The Lord has established his throne in the heavens,
*   and his kingdom rules over all.*
Bless the Lord, O you his angels,
*   you mighty ones who do his bidding,*
*   obedient to his spoken word.*
Bless the Lord, all his hosts,
*   his ministers that do his will.*
Bless the Lord, all his works,
*   in all places of his dominion.*
Bless the Lord, O my soul.

I think biblical David had a really good handle on all the forgiveness that God was willing to dish out. Biblical David (and probably Father David) screw up all the time. And yet God keeps calling the Davids back. And they keep going back because they know it's completely worth it. The Davids (and the Annas) know that their life is infinitely better when God is a part of the equation.

Why do we continue to screw up and constantly need reconciliation and redemption? Wouldn't it be easier if everyone just loved God and loved their neighbor? Isn't that at the root of what Jesus is trying to teach us? I don't have a good or easy answer for any of these questions. We are just human and screw up. It has a lot to do with how feelings, hurts, and injustices happen to us and we want things to be fixed for us. Perhaps God is telling us that a lot of life isn't just about taking care of our individual selves; it's about self-sacrifice in knowing that all will be well with God. This cycle of repentance, penance, redemption, reconciliation, and absolution are all tools to help us get back where we need to be: a life centered on God and not ourselves and our hurts. Again, it's not remotely easy, and as they say "the best things in life are never easy."

What we experience makes us more into people who put God first and not ourselves. Sometimes when we look back at all we've experienced, when we have no explanations or quick fixes to our problems, the only thing that makes a little bit of sense is trusting in something bigger than us. "Trust in God." When I read the psalms and the message behind biblical David's story, I am always reassured and struck that when we don't get it, God does. Our trust in God goes a long way for learning how to live with whatever has happened in our lives.

THOUGHTS TO PONDER

1. What do you worry about that you'll screw up on again?

_____

_____

_____

2. Is it easy or hard for you to "trust in God" ? Why?

_____

_____

_____

3. What would make it easier for you to "trust in God" when nothing else makes sense?

_____

_____

_____

DAY 36   Steps taken: _____   Miles journeyed: _____

Exercise chosen: _____

Something I thought about: _____

_____

_____

_____

_____

Something I need to pray about: _____

_____

_____

_____

_____

Where Is the New Hope, the New Birth, the New Us?

BIBLICAL BIG IDEA #37

For neither circumcision nor uncircumcision is anything; but a new creation is everything! —Galatians 6:15

Me: Hey God?
God: Yes?
Me: I feel kinda old and worn out.
God: How do you think I feel?

During my difficult homecoming from Iraq, I stumbled on the theological work of Paul Tillich. Tillich was a German army chaplain in World War I and was severely traumatized by what he experienced in three of the four major battles of the war. He read the burial service for countless young men, and when his friend, a fellow officer in his unit, died, he could not even read the words on the page. Three times he was MEDIVACed to the rear to recover from combat fatigue, and his bravery under fire earned him the Iron Cross, the highest award in the German army.

He came home to a pregnant wife, although the child was a friend's and not his own. He divorced and crashed hard. But it was during this time that the seeds of his later theological work began to be planted. In the 1930s the Nazis rose to power in Germany and he was the first non-Jewish professor to lose his job. He moved to the United States and began to teach and write theology.

I connect to so much in Tillich's story, albeit my experiences in Iraq paled in comparison to the killing fields of World War I. I read his theology and his biography, trying to make connections between the two. The verse from Paul's letter to the Galatians above was one of his favorites.

He argued that circumcision represented religion in all its bureaucratic splendor and uncircumcision represented the secular atheism that was rapidly rising in Europe and the United States in the 1950s and '60s. From this verse Tillich argued that neither religion or anti-religion can save us. He knew this personally, for the religion that sent him to war failed him and an entire generation of young people. The religion he grew up in was wedded to the nationalistic ideals of the aristocratic German government of the time. Their overconfidence in conquest turned disastrous for millions. Tillich also knew the anti-religion that came in its wake was just as hopeless. He knew he needed something completely different after his traumatic journey.

And so, with Paul, he preached that what we need is a "new creation." We need to find this new creation in Jesus Christ, because he is the new creation. Religion or anti-religion is not enough for traumatized people. What we need is a whole new way of being human.

In our traumas we die, and these deaths give us the opportunity for resurrection. If you've made it this far, I can assure you that resurrection is just around the corner. There are fast and slow resurrections. The resurrection I like to think about is the birth of a new baby. The process takes forever—just ask any mother. And so it is with the new life, the new creation, the new you that comes on the far side of trauma and loss.

THOUGHTS TO PONDER

1. During your time of loss, did you turn to religion? Did you turn to anti-religion? Why?

_____

_____

_____

2. How is Jesus both religious and anti-religious for you?

_____

_____

_____

3. What can we learn from religious and anti-religious people about reconciliation after trauma?

_____

_____

_____

DAY 37 Steps taken: _____ Miles journeyed: _____

Exercise chosen: _____

Something I thought about: _____

_____

_____

_____

_____

Something I need to pray about: _____

_____

_____

_____

_____

38 How Are We Sanctified?

BIBLICAL BIG IDEA #38

*I will rescue you from your people and from the Gentiles—
to whom I am sending you to open their eyes so that they
may turn from darkness to light and from the power of Satan
to God, so that they may receive forgiveness of sins and
a place among those who are sanctified by faith in me.*
—Acts 26:17–18

Me: Hey God?

God: Yes?

Me: I feel unclean. This world makes me dirty, uncomfortable,
and angry.

God: Focus on me and not on the world. The world is not
forever; I am.

The whole reconciliation process includes steps that are sanctifying you
in the eyes of God. As Paul tells us, sanctification is the process in which
we live a life of faith, a life that is focused on God and not the noise of
the world. My disease and all that my body throws at me tells me that
I am "less than." The world tells me that I am "less than" in so many
ways: my body is broken; my fitness doesn't equal six-pack abs and a
four-minute mile; because I believe in the "woo-woo" of something I
cannot see, feel, touch, or hear. The world tells me that my dad is "less
than" because he has a mental illness and all my brothers and sisters that
suffer are "less than" because they haven't met some ideal of perfection
that is espoused by social media, the news, or whatever nonsense a company is trying to sell you. All this noise tells me that I am "less than."
And yet, it is God that tells me that I am worth something.

God tells us that we are made in God's image. We are enough when
we focus on God and our faith. When I walk the path set before me,

I am enough. I am taking care of this world and the people of God by joining in a practice of faith that loves me, loves God, and loves my brothers and sisters. Each step I take towards practicing faith and pushing out the noise that I am "less than" is part of the process of sanctification. When I practice repentance and forgiveness of my sins, I am dedicating myself to God. When I leave behind my pain, ills, anger and discomfort with the world, I am telling and showing the world that my faith is bigger than any belief that I am "less than."

Do you remember the gospel hymn from your childhood, "This Little Light of Mine"?[14]

[Chorus] *This little light of mine, I'm gonna let it shine*
This little light of mine, I'm gonna let it shine
This little light of mine, I'm gonna let it shine
Let it shine, shine, shine
Let it shine!

Everywhere I go, I'm gonna let it shine
Everywhere I go, I'm gonna let it shine
Everywhere I go, I'm gonna let it shine
Let it shine, shine, shine
Let it shine!
[Chorus]

All up in my house, I'm gonna let it shine
All up in my house, I'm gonna let it shine
All up in my house, I'm gonna let it shine
Let it shine, shine, shine
Let it shine!
[Chorus]

Out there in the dark
I'm gonna let it shine
Out there in the dark
I'm gonna let it shine

---

14. John Lomax, 1939.

Out there in the dark
I'm gonna let it shine
Let it shine, shine, shine
Let it shine!
[Chorus]

Sanctification is letting your light shine. Letting your light out despite the darkness. Being a beacon despite being told you are less than. Shining because you have a faith greater than anything that has happened to you. Paul tells us that sanctification is turning from the dark towards the light in your life and letting it shine. As you move forward in this journey, don't let anything put your light out. Someone needs to see it.

THOUGHTS TO PONDER

1. How is your light burning? Strong? Flickering? Is something trying to snuff it out?

_____

_____

_____

2. Are you living a life of faith versus a life of the world? How do you think you are living your life?

_____

_____

_____

3. Do you see a path forward yet or are you still living in the dark and pain of your experience? What do you need to see your way forward?

_____

_____

_____

DAY 38   Steps taken: _____   Miles journeyed: _____

Exercise chosen: _____

Something I thought about: _____

_____

_____

_____

_____

Something I need to pray about: _____

_____

_____

_____

_____

How Do We Accept Absolution and Move On?

BIBLICAL TAKEAWAY #39
"So [the Prodigal Son] set off and went to his father. But while he was still far off, his father saw him and was filled with compassion; he ran and put his arms around him and kissed him." —Luke 15:20

Me: Hey God?
God: Yes?
Me: How will I know when it's time to move on?
God: I hope you never move on.

So much of recovery language is focused on "moving on." With this metaphor, we can imagine the long timeline of our lives, punctuated by trauma and joy, filled in with boredom and monotony. We are moving along this timeline toward our final destiny, and so we put our trauma and sins behind us, hoping we can forget them. If you've stayed with us on this whole journey, you know this is not completely possible. The key to moving on is being able to do what the prodigal son did—he went home. What we often call "moving on" can also be seen as "coming home."

When we move on from our sin, our trauma, that place where we want to escape, we often feel like we are in new territory. We are like the explorers who set out to discover a new land but are inadvertently blown back to their own shoreline. They step ashore and everything is a wonder, a delight. It looks like a new place, because they are new people. When we come home to God our faith is never the same because we are not the same.

We, like the prodigal son, stumble down the country lane we abandoned, wondering what will happen when we reach our father's house. And just as we might collapse in the heat, we hear the footsteps of God coming toward us—and God is coming to us running. God runs to us as we shuffle toward God. God sprints toward us, even when we cannot go another step toward God. The key in this situation is not to run away, not to disappear. God is running at us to kiss us like the father kisses his son who has wasted every gift the father gave him. Can you hear God's footfalls running toward you? Can you feel that kiss on your head and the pull into a bear hug of mercy and grace? If you can't, start this book over or contact Anna or me. Contact your local minister or priest. Reach out to a friend you trust.

Paul Tillich, who I mentioned earlier, often said, "Accept the fact you are accepted." He preached this often because he saw too many people dying inside from all-consuming shame from their past. Lord knows Paul Tillich had plenty himself (see my book on the subject[15]). But even as he preached this message to others, he confessed he had the hardest time preaching it to himself. He had a hard time accepting the fact he was accepted.

Most of us need a combo of means to move on with our lives, to fully realize we have come home. We need other people reminding us of this. We need a faith community that reminds us of this in the general confession and absolution. We need works of art, songs, and poems that remind us of our new reality in Jesus Christ. We also need practices and rituals that remind us of these things. I hope the rituals of walking and running have reminded you that you are accepted and loved. If not, take another lap around the track and ask God to remind you.

---

15. David W. Peters, *Post-Traumatic God: How the Church Cares for People Who Have Been to Hell and Back* (New York: Morehouse, 2016).

THOUGHTS TO PONDER

1. Who is a person in your life who reminds you that you are accepted and forgiven?

_____

_____

_____

2. What ritual do you practice telling yourself you are accepted by God?

_____

_____

_____

DAY 39   Steps taken: _____   Miles journeyed: _____

Exercise chosen: _____

Something I thought about: _____

_____

_____

_____

_____

Something I need to pray about: _____

_____

_____

_____

_____

40 What Actions Do We Take during Absolution?

BIBLICAL BIG IDEA #40

Happy are those whose transgression is forgiven, whose sin is covered. —Psalm 32:1

Me: Hey God?
God: Yes?
Me: I love you.
God: I know.

On this final day in our journey together I want you to know you are absolved, you are forgiven, and you are very much loved. Hopefully you've digested the forgiveness God gives us into your everyday life. You are making steps of faith in all the decisions you make on a daily basis. When we are absolved and living a forgiven life we see faith, hope, and love in all we do. If you take nothing else from the journey you've just taken with David and me, I hope you know these three things. If you take one thing away, I hope you take away the message that you are loved. Just like Paul tells us

And now faith, hope, and love abide, these three; and the greatest of these is love. —1 Corinthians 13:13

We have taken a journey of faith together. I hope that David and I sowed the seeds of hope; we've prayed and loved over these words that we've written so that you will have come to a place where maybe you have or have not reconciled yourself, but at least you've received the message that it's waiting for you. Don't stop walking this journey. Keep tracking your miles, keep moving, and keep praying. God isn't going anywhere. As I believe that God is omnipresent and omniscient, so I believe your time will come and God will be there. God will always love you. Always.

THOUGHTS TO PONDER

1. Do you feel absolved?

_____

_____

_____

2. Will you keep walking these steps of faith?

_____

_____

_____

3. Where do you think your journey will take you next?

_____

_____

4. What I accomplished this 40-day journey:

_____

_____

_____

DAY 40 Steps taken: _____ Miles journeyed: _____

Exercise chosen: _____

Something I thought about: _____

_____

_____

_____

_____

Something I need to pray about: _____

_____

_____

_____

_____

Appendices

Suggested Walking Routes*

Individual and Beginner Routes

Name of Route	Description	Total Distance	Distance Per Day
Nazareth Challenge	The route between Jesus' hometown of Nazareth and Jerusalem	65 miles	1.6 miles or 4,000 steps per day
Jerusalem to Damascus	Paul's conversion on the Damascus Road took place along this journey.	150 miles	3.75 miles or 7,500 steps per day

Intermediate Routes

Name of Route	Description	Total Distance	Distance Per Day
The Jerusalem Challenge	The *Via Dolorosa* (Way of Sorrows) is the route Jesus took through Jerusalem during the last week of his life, which included his preaching in the Temple, clearing the Temple of the money-changers, his Last Supper with the disciples, his arrest in the Garden of Gethsemane, his trial, and his crucifixion.	88 miles	2.2 miles or about 5,500 steps per day
Damascus to Caesarea	One of Paul's missionary journeys	200 miles	5 miles or 10,000 steps per day (a pedometer is recommended)

*All distances are approximate and renditions from maps of the Holy Land.

Advanced

Name of Route	Description	Total Distance	Distance Per Day
The Bethlehem Challenge	The distance between Bethlehem and Jerusalem, representing the beginning and end of Christ's life	200 miles	5 miles or 10,000 steps per day (without using a pedometer)*

*This challenge is done without a fitness tracker. This means that you will get 5 miles of exercise during one workout instead of accumulating the miles over the course of a day with a pedometer.

Name of Route	Description	Total Distance	Distance Per Day
Tarsus to Jerusalem Challenge	One of Paul's missionary journeys	390 miles	9.75 miles of 19,500 steps per day (fitness tracker recommended)
The Exodus Challenge	The route the Israelites traveled to get to the Promised Land of Canaan	375 miles	9.4 miles or 18,750 steps per day (fitness tracker recommended)

Group Challenges

Pool each individual participant's miles each week to reach a group distance goal.

Name of Route	Description	Total Distance	Distance Per Day
The Abraham Migration	Represents Abraham's wanderings to find the Promised Land to begin the birth of God's people	900 miles	22.5 miles per day
Jerusalem to Antioch (round trip)	One of Paul's missionary journeys	705 miles	17.25 miles per day
Paul's First Missionary Journey	Paul's first mission trip	1,300 miles	32.5 miles per day
Ephesus to Jerusalem	One of Paul's missionary trips	800 miles	20 miles per day
Jerusalem to Rome	The end of the road for Paul	1,800 miles	45 miles per day

Group Challenges (continued)

Name of Route	Description	Total Distance	Distance Per Day
Jerusalem to Corinth	One of Paul's missionary journeys	1,050 miles	26.25 miles per day
Antioch to Philippi	A portion of Paul's third missionary journey	950 miles	23.75 miles per day

Beginner Walks

Nazareth Challenge: It is 65 miles between Jesus' hometown of Nazareth and Jerusalem. This is approximately 1.6 miles each day for forty days to walk the distance of the route that Jesus preached to reach his end in Jerusalem. Set a goal to walk 1.6 miles each day or 4,000 steps per day during Lent (or any forty day period of your choosing), or complete 65 miles by the end of the six-week period.

Jerusalem to Damascus: This journey represents Paul's conversion on the Damascus Road. It is 150 miles or 3.75 miles per day or 7,500 steps a day.

Intermediate Walks

Jerusalem Challenge: During Jesus' final days, his route through Jerusalem included preaching at the Temple, clearing the Temple of the money changers, the last supper with his disciples, his arrest in the Garden of Gethsemane, his trial, Peter's denial, and his crucifixion. This route was approximately 2.2 miles in length. Set a goal to walk 2.2 miles each day during Lent, or about 5,500 steps per day.

Damascus to Caesarea: One of Paul's missionary journeys was about 200 miles or 5 miles per day or 10,000 steps a day. You can use a pedometer throughout the day to accumulate the miles.

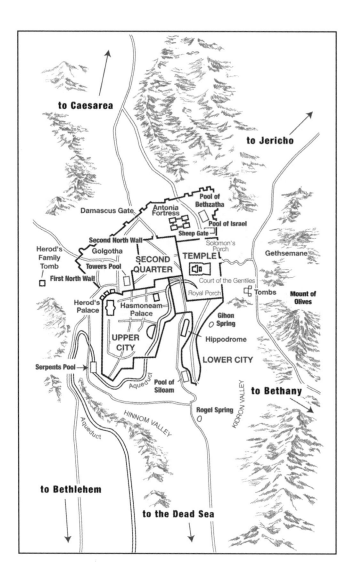

Advanced Walks

Bethlehem Challenge: It is five miles between Bethlehem and Jerusalem. This represents the beginning to the end of Christ's journey. Set a goal to walk five miles without using a pedometer.

Tarsus to Jerusalem: This is Paul's route from his home town of Tarsus to Jerusalem. 390 miles or 9.75 miles a day or 19,500 steps a day

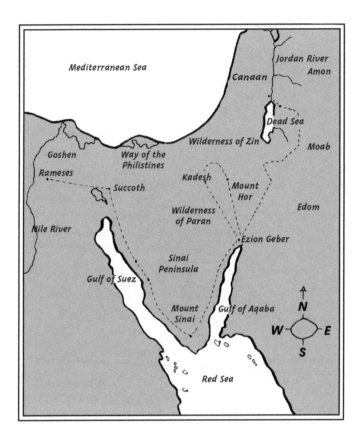

The Exodus: The route the Israelites traveled to get to the Promised Land is 375 miles, 9.4 miles per day or 18,750 steps per day. (This may be used as a group challenge.)

Group Challenges

These goals should be divided based on the number of people in your group and how many miles each group member will commit to walking during the forty-day challenge:

The Abraham Migration: This represents Abraham's wanderings to find the Promised Land to begin the birth of God's people. It is roughly 900 miles, or 22.5 miles a day.

Jerusalem to Antioch: This is the first part of Paul's second missionary journey. Paul was preaching to the Gentiles in Antioch. This was one of the first times in which God's word was shared to other Christians not of Jewish descent. This is a round trip of 705 miles or 17.25 miles a day.

Antioch to Cyprus: This is part of Paul's 1st missionary journey. Paul and Barnabas travel from Antioch to Barnabas' home in Salamis, Cyprus to preach the word of God. 1,300 miles or 32.5 miles a day

Ephesus to Jerusalem: This is a portion of Paul's third missionary journey. The Letter to the Ephesians is one of Paul's most famous letters written while building the church in the city of Ephesus. The church later became one of the heads of the seven churches of Asia Minor and contributed to the spread of Christianity across what is modern day Turkey. 800 miles or 20 miles a day

Paul's Journey to Rome: Paul's journey from Jerusalem to Rome where he finally died for his beliefs. It is said that Paul's body is buried underneath St. Paul's Cathedral in Vatican City. 1,800 miles or 45 miles a day

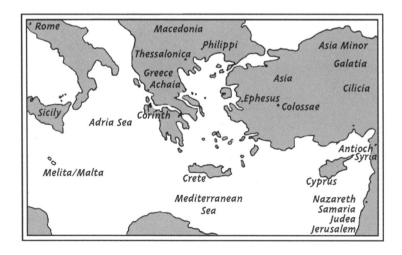

Jerusalem to Corinth: The full route of Paul's third missionary journey to Corinth, Greece. Paul is the founder of the Christian church in Corinth. In his letter to the Corinthians, Paul gives thanks for his health, his journey, his deliverance from dangers, and for the people of Corinth. 1050 miles or 26.25 miles a day

Antioch to Philippi: This is a portion of Paul's 3rd Missionary Journey. The church in Philippi is the first Christian church founded by Paul in Europe. 950 miles or 23.75 miles a day

Fitness Tracker Usage and Mileage Calculations

We strongly encourage you to use a fitness tracker (FitBit, Garmen, Fitness tracker, Omron, etc.) to monitor the steps and miles you accumulate towards your Biblical Walking Goal. Roughly 2,000 steps equal a mile on your fitness tracker and most trackers will calculate this for you. Steps and mileage calculation depend on the length of your stride and the accuracy of your miles will depend on the sophistication of your fitness tracker. This isn't meant to be a punitive journey though, so if you think your fitness tracker is cheating your steps or miles, track what is the most accurate and truthful representation of your miles on your journey.

You do not have to walk; you can use a treadmill, run, bike, swim or whatever activity you choose to do. Approximately fifteen minutes of physical activity will equal a mile if you are unable to calculate the mileage. (For example, fifteen minutes of an aerobics/yoga class would be a mile for the purpose of this program.)

If you are unable to walk, consider using each fifteen-minute block in volunteering or in prayer. Our goal is to transform spiritually as well as physically. There are no penalties in *Christ Walk Crushed*! Focus on things you can do to change your life through increased activity, or increased prayer, or increased work for others. Use your fitness tracker all day so that *all* of your activity will be included towards your goal. Please join us in a journey taking a step of faith in Christ.

Mileage Calculation Chart

Activity	Time	Steps	Record Miles As:
Walking	15–20 minutes	2,000–2,500	1 or distance on route
Running	Varies	2,000–2,500	Check route distance
Biking	Varies	N/A	Check odometer distance
Aerobics	15 minutes	Varies	1
Dancing	15 minutes	Varies	1
Yoga	15 minutes	Varies	1
Prayer/Meditation	15 minutes	Varies	1
Volunteerism	15 minutes	Varies	1

A Few Healthy Eating and Exercise Habits

HEALTHY EATING

- Eat slowly and at a table
- Limit distractions like TV, phone, news (*This allows you to enjoy the food you're eating and makes you more aware of what you're eating.*)
- Eat regular meals and plan snacks (*This allows you to stay in control of eating and increases metabolic rate.*)
- Exercise three to five times a week
- Enjoy eating
- Relax and slow down (*It takes twenty minutes for the brain to know you are full. Eating fast leads to excessive eating.*)
- Drink liquids between bites
- Set down utensils (spoon/chopsticks)
- Chew and savor food while you eat
- *Enjoy* sharing meal time

TIPS TO SPEED UP YOUR METABOLISM

- Quit starving yourself
- Start exercising
- Exercise longer
- Exercise large muscle groups
- Vary your workout

SETTING REALISTIC EXERCISE GOALS

- Walk to work
- Exercise (sit-ups, push-ups, jumping jacks, etc.) in front of the TV
- Walk during lunch hour
- Walk instead of driving whenever you can
- Take a family walk after dinner
- Mow your lawn with a push mower
- Walk to your place of worship instead of driving
- Walk your kids to school
- Join an exercise group
- Replace Sunday drive with Sunday walk
- Incorporate ten minutes of exercise, three times a day into your routine instead of trying to do it all at once.

SUPPORTING YOUR GOALS

- For the most part, we control our environment
- Are you taking extra steps every day to increase physical activity in your life?
- Are you making healthy choices?
- It's not about punishment and denial, it's about good choices
- Change is difficult, even if it's about small choices
- Consistency: The #1 key to success
  - The more you exercise, the easier it gets
  - When all else fails, keep going
  - The more frequently you make healthy food choices, the easier it gets

OTHER STICK-TO STRATEGIES

- Use a fitness tracker
- Christ Walk Crush!
- Get a dog!

- Leave yourself exercise reminders like setting your walking shoes out for your morning walk before you go to bed
- Clean your pantry of temptations! (Would you keep the devil in your back pocket?)
- Make sure you are having fun with whatever you choose to do!

Suggestions for Groups

Christ Walk Crushed was intended to be a group activity. People who have communities of wellness are more likely to be successful in their goals. Teams are successful when they:

- Meet together

- Exercise together

- Pray together

- Share successes and challenges together

- Encourage each other

If you are not experiencing *Christ Walk Crushed* as a part of a church educational or devotional period, try to get a group of friends together to experience the lessons and activities together. Your Bible study, men's, or women's group can complete *Christ Walk Crushed*. The purpose is to commit to improving your health together as you help each other along to a healthier you. If you do not have access to a group, join a virtual team through Fitbit, Facebook, or other group so that you are not alone in your journey.

Christ Walk™ can be found online at:

- Facebook: www.facebook.com/christwalk40day

- Twitter: @christwalk1

- Blog: www.blogspot.christwalk40day.com

- Instagram: @christwalk1

Another suggestion for groups is to invite a fitness professional to discuss principles of fitness as a special guest. I also recommend a fitness professional come to conduct fitness testing with each individual followed by individualized fitness plan recommendations based on the results of the fitness test for everyone.

Suggestions for Group Leaders

If you are taking on the role as a *Christ Walk Crushed* group leader, congratulations! What an awesome experience for you and your team or church. You can join the *Christ Walk Crushed* forum on Facebook to discuss ideas and goals with members of the *Christ Walk Crushed* community around the globe! I am happy to provide feedback or guidance on running a group *Christ Walk Crushed*. *Christ Walk Crushed* can be found online at:

- Facebook: www.facebook.com/christwalk40day
- Twitter: @christwalk1
- Blog: www.blogspot.christwalk40day.com
- Instagram: @christwalk1

The number one guidance I offer in leading *Christ Walk Crushed* is to give freely of yourself and your experience. You may have a lot of fitness experience or none at all, but since we all have health, we all have a perspective that can be shared and discussed in our small-group settings that are valuable to anyone in the room. I have led groups from as few as five participants to as many as eighty, and the experience can be as much as we choose to share with each other during our time together. Give freely of yourself and your experience. This builds a bond of a shared experience.

There are several ways that the *Christ Walk Crushed* experience can be structured for groups:

- As a simple Bible study, meet each week to discuss the "Thoughts to Ponder" after each day's reading. Simply share your experiences with those meditations. Make sure that everyone reports and tracks their miles to their destination.

- Meet each week to focus on a different topic (See Appendix F for an outline):
  - Week One: Introduction
  - Week Two: Physical Health
  - Week Three: Mental Health
  - Week Four: Spiritual Health
  - Week Five: Nutrition
  - Week Six: Pot Luck and Graduation/Sharing
- Meet each week to discuss one of the scripture readings from the meditations, sharing what each says to the members of your group about their health, spirituality, or moral injury.
- Meet each week and have a theological reflection on one of the topics on the week's readings. Discuss the topic from the point of view of creation, sin, judgment, repentance, and redemption. (See Appendix F for an outline.)
  - Week One: Introduction
  - Week Two: Creation—How is God creating something new in us?
  - Week Three: Sin—Where have we gone wrong?
  - Week Four: Judgment—Where are we caught up short?
  - Week Five: Repentance—Where have we sought forgiveness?
  - Week Six: Redemption—Where have we been forgiven?
- Meet each week and provide keys to healthy living.
  - Week One: Introduction
  - Week Two: Health Fair/Health Assessment
  - Week Three: Making Change/Change Exercise/Goal Setting
  - Week Four: Fitness Testing
  - Week Five: Cooking Classes
  - Week Six: Healthy Potluck

Need other Ideas? Join me on Facebook, Twitter, or the blog for a discussion of group options. I am happy to answer questions as they are posted!

Happy Christ Walking!

Christ Walk Crushed Program Outlines

Christ Walk makes a perfect program for adults (or youth) who desire to improve or change their habits toward a healthier life—body, mind, and spirit. Each week correlates to a section of *Christ Walk Crushed* (the book), and each participant should have a copy for recording their progress in the journal sections.

Options

- Day or evening sessions: 1 hour
- Evenings with a meal and worship: 2.5 hours
  - Pot Luck meal—1 hour
  - Session—1 hour
  - Compline or Evening Prayer—30 minutes
- Session with a meal: 2 hours
  - Potluck meal—1 hour
  - Session—1 hour

Two models are offered here for holding your own *Christ Walk Crushed* program in your church, organization, or with friends. Feel free to mix them together, substitute your own activities, or adapt to create your own program. Consider offering childcare during the sessions, or holding a children's program concurrent with the adult program. It is never too early to help our children build healthy habits for body, mind, and spirit! Try *Christ Walk Kids* as part of your youth program.

Useful Materials

It is useful to have a number of materials available for the class meeting times. A list of tools I have on hand when I lead a *Christ Walk Crushed* group include:

- A computer and projector with any PowerPoint presentations you may use to help with the weekly discussions
- Poster board or newsprint (with markers) for the teams to use for the activity
- Newsprint, easel, and tape for the leader to write up brainstorming comments and important discussion points
- A poster of all the team names and routes chosen (You can have them add up their miles each week and put it on their team poster.)

Publicity

When organizing a class, make sure to spread the word using your church's newsletter, weekly bulletin, website, Facebook page, or even the local newspaper. Here are two samples you can adapt.

Newsletter article sample #1

Have you ever wondered what it would have been like to walk with Jesus? There were no cars two thousand years ago. Jesus walked throughout his ministry. The *Christ Walk Crushed* program allows us to walk the miles of various routes in the Bible during the next forty days. Walking is a very holy activity that almost anyone can do at any fitness level. The benefits of walking are numerous for every age. Some of the routes that we can explore include the *Via Dolorosa* (Christ's last walk through Jerusalem), the Nazareth-Jerusalem route, Paul's missionary journeys, the spread of Christianity from Jerusalem to Rome, and many more. I invite you to join us on a journey of a lifetime as we study mind, body, and spiritual health through the process of reconciliation with *Christ Walk Crushed.*

The *Christ Walk Crushed* program will be offered at (*insert your church/address*) beginning on (*insert dates and times*) as a forty-day mind, body, and spiritual wellness program for Lent (*or any other season or timeframe*). Individuals and teams will select various routes of the Bible and count steps or miles towards their goal. Each week we will meet in fellowship to have a program on a different aspect of mind, body, and spiritual health. Teams will participate in reflective exercises that will help them grow towards a Christ-centered life. Every aspect of what we do can be lifted as an offering to God, even taking care of our bodies. There is a "God-spark" in each of us and our bodies are the temple that God gives us to explore our gifts and talents. Taking care of that body to do God's work is paramount.

If you are interested in *Christ Walk Crushed*, or would like more information on the program, please contact (*insert contact information*). *Christ Walk Crushed* is available to anyone at any fitness level. A participant even walked her routes with her walker! You can experience *Christ Walk Crushed*, too. Peace and happy trails, (*your name*).

Newsletter article sample #2

An amazing thing will happen this Lent (*or other forty-day/6 week period*) at church! We will get to exercise and eat at the same time! Study Suppers return with various groups within the church catering a lovely dinner of soup and salad each Wednesday (*or other day*) at 6:00 p.m. in the Parish Hall. Dinner will be followed by the *Christ Walk Crushed* program, a forty-day walking program than encompasses mind, body, and spiritual health during the forty days of Lent.

- Week 1: Introduction and goal-setting
- Week 2: (insert topic)
- Week 3: (insert topic)
- Week 4: (insert topic)
- Week 5: (insert topic)
- Week 6: Healthy potluck and graduation (optional)

Childcare will be available and there will be a special youth team option. Join us starting (*insert date*) at (*insert time*) in the Parish Hall. There will be a sign-up sheet in the church so that we can ensure there are enough materials for everyone interested in participating. The program is open to all, no matter your health or fitness level. If you have questions, feel free to contact (*insert contact name*) via (*email*) or (*phone*). See you on the journey!

Ice Breakers

ICE BREAKER A: INTRODUCE A NEW FRIEND

- Pair up with someone you do not know
- Ask them to take one to three things from their wallet, purse, pocket, etc., and use those three things to describe themselves
- Introduce your partner to the group

ICE BREAKER B: FORMING TEAMS

- Pair up with someone you do not know
- Ask each other questions until you find something you have in common
- Go find another team you do not know—talk to each other until you find something all four of you have in common
- Do this one more time until you have a group of six (or four to five, depending on group totals: You are building your walking teams with this method.)
- Choose a group speaker who tells the larger group what you all have in common
- Look closely at the people in your group
- This is your Christ Walk Crushed team!
- Pray for each other!

ICE BREAKER C: BIBLE STUDY

This can also serve as the introduction to the program as you move into the leader discussion points.

- "And this is love, that we walk according to his commandments; this is the commandment just as you have heard from the beginning—you must walk in it." 2 John 1:6
- What does walking in love mean? Discuss in small groups.
- Share with the larger group
- Leader points that can be shared:
  - We are called to walk with Christ in our everyday life
  - We can use the Holy Spirit to work towards better mind, body, and spiritual health

- We walk to do God's work
- We walk to make our bodies stronger to do God's work
- We pray to do God's work
- Our mind, body, and spiritual health are for us to do God's work
- *Christ Walk Crushed* is. . . the journey of making our bodies stronger, mind, body, and spirit, to DO God's work for all of our lives

Example 1
Walking with Christ: A Five- or Six-Week Program

Week 1: Introducing *Christ Walk Crushed*

Week 2: Christ Calls Us to Change

Week 3: What is Health? A Group Reflection on the Definition of Health

Week 4: Meditation and Health *or* Nutrition and Health

Week 5: Where Do I Go From Here? Keeping the Journey Going

Week 6: Healthy Potluck (optional)

Week 1: Introducing Christ Walk Crushed
Gather

Open with Prayer
You can assign weekly prayer duties to each of the teams in your group if you have a large enough group, or ask volunteers to lead opening and closing prayer each week.

Introduce an Ice Breaker

Presentation and Discussion

Leader's Talking Points

- We are called to walk with Christ in our everyday life

- Mind, body, and spirit

- Each day we should resolve to walk with Christ

- We can use the Holy Spirit to work towards better mind, body, and spiritual health

We'll be using the actual motion of "walking with Christ" during this challenge and goal towards better mind, body, and spiritual health. This goal will be a metaphor for many changes in our lives and how we are called to serve Christ, how we stick with it, how we might slip up, and how we take this on to the rest of our lives.

- With this challenge you begin your commitment to walk with Christ.

- You will choose a walking challenge to work on during Lent (or whatever time frame you have chosen).

- You can choose to pair up with a buddy to work together towards your walk with Christ.

- You will choose an individual goal and your group will choose a group goal. (This is a good time to distribute the *Christ Walk Crushed* books and check out the appendices.)

- There is room in the back of your book to track your daily miles towards your goal.

- Each day in your book includes journal space to help you on your way:
  - Spaces to record distance
  - Spaces to record reflective thoughts on journey
  - Daily prayers and thoughts on a Christ-centered life

Considerations for Walking

- You may use a pedometer (step counter) to measure your distance each day. Approximately 2,000 to 2,500 steps equals 1 mile. (Option: Distribute pedometers to each participant.)

- You do not have to walk; you can use a treadmill, run, bike, swim, or whatever activity you can measure in terms of miles.

- If you cannot measure mileage, roughly fifteen minutes of physical activity (like an aerobics class) equals one mile. The important thing is to choose something to be physically active.

- Document miles in mile tracker in *Christ Walk Crushed*—there is a table in the back of the book to use *(see page 202)*.

- If you get a pedometer or a Fitbit or other fitness-tracking device, (available at places like Target, Wal-Mart or any other sporting goods store), we can discuss use at the next class. Otherwise, start keeping track of the steps and miles you are taking with your new fitness tracker.

Activity: Your Walking Team

- Break into team(s)
- Brainstorm team name
- Develop short team prayer
- Agree on team walking goal
- Share with the larger group

Conclusion

Wrap-Up

- Review mind, body, and spiritual journey
- Develop a Christ-centered life through mind, body, and spiritual exercises (exercise, study, eat good food, pray and/or meditate!)
- Questions?

Homework

- Choose a walking challenge
- Meditate on the purpose of your goal and the change you want to happen in the next six weeks
- Purchase pedometer, or Fitbit, or other fitness tracker
- Pray for your team

Close with Prayer

Week 2: Christ Calls Us to Change
Gather
Open with Prayer

Presentation and Discussion
Leader's Talking Points

- We've committed to a mind, body, and spiritual journey towards total well-being
- You have begun your physical walk with Christ
- Let's discuss how Christ calls us to change our lives to be more Christ-centered
- Discuss the Change Exercise (below) and the three most important things in your life

Activity: "Christ Calls Us to Change" Exercise
Distribute paper and pencils to each participant. Directions:

- Write your name
- Write the most important things in your life under your name
- Turn the piece of paper over and write one thing that you would like to change or work on during Lent (or whatever time frame you are following)
- How does the thing you want to change about yourself reflect on what you say are the most important things in your life?
- Is God one of the most important things in your life?
- How does your habit reflect on your relationship with God?
- Can you use your relationship with God to help you work on what you want to change?

Open the floor to discussion or questions. Ask if anyone wants to share his or her own personal goal to change. Volunteer what you want to change about yourself. Give freely of your experience.

Let's brainstorm how we can use God to work on mind, body, and spiritual well-being to help us change. Note these on newsprint.

Goal Discussion:
Leader's Talking Points:

- Giving up chocolate, caffeine, alcohol, sweets, meat, etc.
- Taking on readings, mission work, prayer
- Results in self-discipline and spiritual discipline especially if you use prayer and the Holy Spirit as your source of strength towards giving up indulgences

Conclusion

Wrap-Up

- What did you decide you wanted to change for this challenge?
- What are some tools that you have to support you through this?
- Do the three most important things in your life support what you want to change?
- If not, do you need to rethink the most important things in your life?
- Questions? Thoughts?

Close with Prayer

Week 3: Group Discussion: What is Health?

Gather

Open with Prayer

Presentation and Discussion

Leader's Talking Points

Taking care of our body is like taking care of Christ as we are made in his image. A whole and healthy body is a body that can be more devoted to his call in your life.

The World Health Organization's definition of health: "Health is a state of complete physical, mental, and social wellbeing and not merely the absence of disease or infirmity."

Activity: What Does Health Look Like?

Leader's Talking Points:

Print the above definition on newsprint and record your conversation on the following for all to see:

- Step One: Let's discuss the definition:
  - What stands out in the statement?
  - What do you know about the statement?
  - What is happening in the text?
  - What kind of text is this?

- Step Two: What does the Bible say?
  - What is the world like in this passage?
  - What human predicament is revealed?
  - What indicates a change of mind, heart, or behavior?
  - What gives celebration for the world?
  - What does the Bible or church tradition say about health?

- Step Three: What does your own experience say about this?
  - How do you identify with this passage?
  - Can you recall a time in your life where you felt or did not feel this way?
  - What are your thoughts and feelings on this definition?
  - What does your health mean to you in light of our conversation?
  - In what way does your faith support, inform, or challenge you in light of this definition?

- Step Four: What does our culture (the world around us) say about health?

- Step Five: What is your position on health?
  - Where do you stand?
  - "I believe. . . ."

- Step Six: Insights and Implications

Conclusion

Wrap-Up
Leader's Talking Points:

- How's your walking going?
- What goals will you make to become healthier?

Close with Prayer

Week 4: *Meditation and Health or Nutrition and Health*

Gather

Open with Prayer

Presentation and Discussion

Activity Choice A: Meditation and Health
Leader's Talking Points:
Facilitate a period of meditation or walk a labyrinth for this week's activity. Discuss the group's experience.

Activity Choice B: Nutrition and Health: Meals with Jesus
Leader's Talking Points:
Discuss the joy of food. Discuss that Jesus is always eating and drinking in the Bible. There is prayer at the table. There is laughter, and tears, and talking. They are sitting down and they are devoted to one another. No one is eating meal replacement bars or drinks. They are eating real food and they are thrilled to be at Jesus' table. If you have a health background, discuss what healthy eating means. Eat real food, in moderation and with joy.

- Give each group a poster board or newsprint. Have them discuss as a group a menu they would prepare for Jesus.
- Ask each group to share their meal with the larger group and tell WHY they chose this menu to share with Jesus.
- How would it feel to eat a meal with Jesus? What would it mean to you?
- As a group, name foods or meals that occur in the Bible. What do you think about the different biblical meals and the food that God gives us in the Bible?

Conclusion

Wrap-Up

- Thoughts?
- Questions?

Close with Prayer

Week 5: Where Do We Go From Here?

Gather

Open with Prayer

Presentation and Discussion

Activity: Slipping-Up Discussion
Leader's Talking Points

- Throughout your life, when you gave something up, did you make your goal?

- Have you stuck to your walking challenge? Did you meet your goals?

- How has it felt to walk with Christ?

- Is it hard? Christ's life was hard.

- So what? What do we do when we slip up?

Let's brainstorm some ideas of what we can do when we slip up:

- Get back on the wagon
- Pray
- Ask forgiveness
- Reevaluate your goals—are they unattainable? Is it really what Christ is calling you to do?
- Other ways to improve self-discipline
- Stick with your *Christ Walk Crushed* buddies and continue these healthy practices throughout the year, not just during Lent or this study. Encourage each other on each person's journey to healthier life. We each make each other better Christians.

Conclusion

Wrap-Up

- Give thanks to God for the opportunity each day to improve our well-being
- Questions?
- Don't forget to keep plugging away with miles!
- Thank you! Good Luck!

Close with Prayer

Week 6: Conclusion/Graduation/Healthy Potluck (optional):

Host a healthy potluck and challenge your participants to bring a healthy dish and recipe to share.

- Give thanks to God for the opportunity each day to improve our well-being
- Recap the last five weeks.
- Offer the opportunity to share experiences
- Questions?
- Don't forget to keep plugging away with miles!
- Thank you! Good Luck!
- Awards (optional): You can make up awards, get water bottles with your church logo or t-shirts depending on your budget, and give to the participants. You can also create a satisfaction survey if you would like.

Example 2
Walking with Christ: A Six-Week Program of Theological Reflection

Week 1: Introducing Christ Walk Crushed

Week 2: Creation and the Body

Week 3: Sin and the Body

Week 4: Judgment and the Body

Week 5: Repentance and the Body

Week 6: Redemption and the Body

Week 1: Introducing Christ Walk Crushed
Gather

Open with Prayer
You can assign weekly prayer duties to each of the teams in your group if you have a large enough group, or ask volunteers to lead opening and closing prayer each week.

Introduce an Ice Breaker

Presentation and Discussion

Leader's Talking Points:

- We are called to walk with Christ in our everyday life

- Mind, body, and spirit

- Each day we should resolve to walk with Christ

- "This is the day that the Lord has made, let us rejoice and be glad in it."

- We can use the Holy Spirit to work towards better mind, body, and spiritual health

We'll be using the actual motion of "walking with Christ" during this challenge and goal towards better mind, body, and spiritual health. This goal will be a metaphor for many changes in our lives and how we are called to serve Christ, how we stick with it, how we might slip up, and how we take this on to the rest of our lives.

With this challenge you begin your commitment to walk with Christ.

- You will choose a walking challenge to work on during Lent (or whatever time frame you have chosen).

- You can choose to pair up with a buddy to work together towards your walk with Christ.

- You will choose an individual goal and your group will choose a group goal. (This is a good time to distribute the Christ Walk Crushed books and check out the appendices.)

- There is room in the back of your book to track your daily miles towards your goal.

- Each day in your book includes a journal space to help you on your way:
  ○ Spaces to record distance
  ○ Spaces to record reflective thoughts on journey
  ○ Daily prayers and thoughts on a Christ-centered life

Considerations for Walking

- You may use a pedometer (step counter) to measure your distance each day. Approximately 2,000 to 2,500 steps equals 1 mile. (Option: Distribute pedometers to each participant.)

- You do not have to walk; you can use a treadmill, run, bike, swim, or whatever activity you can measure in terms of miles.

- If you cannot measure mileage, roughly fifteen minutes of physical activity (like an aerobics class) equals one mile. The important thing is to choose something to be physically active.

- Document miles in mile tracker in Christ Walk Crushed—there is a table in the back of the book to use *(see page 202)*.

- If you get a pedometer or a Fitbit or other fitness-tracking device (available at places like Target, Wal-Mart or any other sporting goods store), we can discuss use at the next class. Otherwise, start keeping track of the steps and miles you are taking with your new fitness tracker.

Activity: Your Walking Team

- Break into team(s)
- Brainstorm team name
- Develop short team prayer
- Agree on team walking goal
- Share with the larger group

Conclusion

Wrap-Up:

- Review mind, body, and spiritual journey
- Develop a Christ-centered life through mind, body, and spiritual exercises (exercise, study, healthy eating, prayer and/or meditation!)
- Questions?

Homework:

- Choose a walking challenge
- Meditate on the purpose of your goal and the change you want to happen in the next six weeks
- Purchase pedometer, or Fitbit, or other fitness tracker
- Pray for your team

Close with Prayer

Week 2: Creation and the Body

Gather

Open with Prayer

Presentation and Discussion

Leader's Talking Points

- What does society say about creation? How does the secular world define creation?
- What does the church/tradition say about creation? How did God create us?
- What are our conflicts about these two, possibly opposing, views?
- What insights have we had from this discussion?

Use newsprint to capture people's comments/notes. Make a quad chart on the paper:

- In upper right corner write: Society
- In the upper left corner write: Church/Tradition
- In the lower right corner write: What is the conflict between these two beliefs about creation?
- In the lower left corner write: Conclusions/Insights

Facilitate a group discussion of what creation means based on these four different aspects of creation.

Conclusion

Close with Prayer

Week 3: Sin and the Body

Gather

Open with Prayer

Presentation and Discussion

Leader's Talking Points

- What is sin?
- What does sin look like?
- How do we sin in regards to our health?
- What does the Bible say about sin?
- What does society say about sin?
- How does this make us feel?
- Do we feel connected between our physical health and our spiritual health?
- Do we consider our health habits sins?

Method 1: Open a discussion using the questions above and facilitate a conversation using these questions. You can capture thoughts and feelings and consensus from the group on your presentation paper. Close with any insights and comments.

Method 2: Use the Quad Chart method from "Creation." In each corner write:

- What does sin look like?
- What does society say about sin and the body?
- Do we consider our health habits sins?
- How do we feel about this?
- Capture the participants' comments in each quadrant of the chart.
- Close with any final comments and insights.

Conclusion

Close with Prayer

Week 4: Judgment and the Body

Gather

Open with Prayer

Presentation and Discussion

Leader's Talking Points

What is judgment?

- What are the differences between biblical judgment and social judgment? (You can split newsprint in two columns: One with a heading of "biblical judgment" and the other with "social judgment." Capture the participants' comments. See where the discussion leads and then draw the group around to the next topic.

- Do you feel that poor health is an example of judgment?

- Why or why not? (You can use the column method above and discuss why or why not poor health is an example of judgment.) It is very important to facilitate this carefully and nonjudgmentally, reminding the group that everyone's feelings and thoughts are important. Not everyone will agree about this topic. Discuss it lovingly and kindly and remind the group that no one person is correct.

- How does judgment make you feel about God?

- How do we move away from judgment or accept judgment in our lives?

Conclusion

Leader's Talking Points

- Pray about judgment in your life!
- What comes after judgment? Repentance!
- Pray, walk, record/journal, and move!

Close with Prayer

Week 5: Repentance and the Body

Gather

Open with Prayer

Presentation and Discussion

Leader's Talking Points

You may choose to capture the comments on newsprint. This often helps people gain insights from the discussion.

- Recap what we have discovered about our health so far.
- What does repentance mean to you?
- What does repentance of our health habits mean?
- How is that tied to a godly life? Why should what we do physically matter to our spiritual wellness?
- Does it matter?
- How do we show that we are repentant?
- Do you think God cares what we eat, whether we exercise, or if we have healthy habits?
- It is important to realize that the choices you make today will largely determine how healthy you are tomorrow.

Conclusion

Close with Prayer

Week 6: Redemption and the Body

Gather

Open with Prayer

Presentation and Discussion

Leader's Talking Points

Divide a sheet of newsprint in two columns. In one column write: What is redemption of the body? In another column write: What is redemption of the soul? Compare and contrast. Capture insights and similarities on another piece of paper. Other questions for consideration:

- Do you feel you are redeemed?

- Do you feel you are worthy of redemption?

- Do you feel that your health habits lead to a healthier spiritual life?

- Where do we go from here on this journey?

- How do we share our message of redemption, body, mind, and soul, with others?

Conclusion

Close with Prayer

Bibliography

Bachman, Keith L. "Obesity, Weight Management, and Health Care Costs: A Primer." *Disease Management*. 10:3 (2007): 129–137.

Bowman, Shanthy A. "Television-Viewing Characteristics of Adults: Correlations to Eating Practices and Overweight and Health Status," *Preventing Chronic Disease*, 3:2 (2006), 1–11. Accessed on January 29, 2008 from www.cdc.gov/pcd/issues/2006/apr/05_0139.htm.

Green, Beverly B., Allen Cheadle, Adam S. Pellegrini, and Jeffrey Harris. "Active for Life: A Work Based Physical Activity Program. "*Preventing Chronic Disease*" (2007). Accessed on June 18, 2007 from http://www.cdc.gov/pcd/issues/2007/jul/06_0065.htm.

Isaacs, A.J., J.A. Critchley, S.S.Tai, K. Buckingham, D. Westley, S.D.R. Harridge, C. Smith, and J.M. Gottlieb. "Exercise Evaluation Randomized Trial (EXERT): A Randomized trial comparing GP referral for leisure centre-based exercise, community-based walking and advice only." *Health Technology Assessment*. 11:10 (2007), 1–185.

Jakicic, J.M., and A.D. Otto. "Motivating Change: Modifying Eating and Exercise Behaviors for Weight Management." *American College of Sports Medicine Health and Fitness Journal*, 9:1 (2005), 6–12.

Musich, S., T. McDonald, D. Hirschland, and D. Edington. "Examination of Risk Status Transitions Among Active Employees in a Comprehensive Worksite Health Promotion Program." *Journal of Occupational and Environmental Medicine*. 45:4 (2003), 393–399.

Polascsek M., L.M. O'Brien, W. Lagasse, and N. Hammar. "Move & Improve: a worksite wellness program in Maine." *Prevention of Chronic Disease* (2006). Accessed on June 18, 2007 from http://www.cdc.gov/pcd/issues/2006/jul/05_0123.htm.

Samuelson, M. "Stages of change: From theory to practice." *The Art of Health Promotion* 2: 5 (1998): 1–12.

Steps and Mileage Tracker

You can use the following space to track your progress through your challenge. Each day, add in your steps for the day, the miles for the day, and then add that into the total column for a running total of your progress. You can also make copies of these pages to use in subsequent challenges! Enjoy your journey!

Date	Steps	Miles	Today's Total	Running Total

Date	Steps	Miles	Today's Total	Running Total